"In a world that seems to pull us toward an unnatural lifestyle, Bernie's book is a most welcome call to show us that nature really does know best."
James Earls, author of *Born to Walk* and *Understanding the Human Foot* (UK)

"This book will support newborn parents, carers, teachers, and those in the sports, massage and yoga industries who work with babies and children. A great interactive book that got me doing something physical so I could feel what was going on."
P-J McCrea, founder of Little Steps. Beautiful Beginnings (NZ)

"Wow! As a teacher, education researcher and first 1000 days specialist, I had NO idea how important the foot was in the development of the child! I really recommend that every educator reads this fount of fascinating information. For every parent just starting their parenting journey, this will make fascinating reading during your pregnancy and early days. Not only will you learn heaps but you will be so much more informed of ways to support your child in their development from the earliest of days, which in turn will help them to develop to their full. This is like no other pregnancy book!"
Clare Stead, creator and founder of the Oliiki app (UK)

"This is a very valuable book for parents, especially fathers. From personal experience, (new) fathers are sometimes a bit lost as to what they can do with their baby when they have to tend to them. The information and exercises are great way for fathers to do something that is fun as well as helpful! All dads should read this book!"
Gert Lippens, chiropractor and father (UK)

"An inspiring and informative read for parents and those who work with infants. As a midwife I recommend this book to other midwives so they can share this valuable advice with women in their care. *Finding Their Feet* gives practical and well-founded advice on how a parent/caregiver can, with confidence, have an active role in their child's development."

**Dr Heather Donald, midwifery lecturer and researcher,
Auckland University of Technology (NZ)**

"Bernie has really done her research magnificently, and shone the light on the importance of primitive reflexes in the development of the whole nervous system. I recommend *Finding Their Feet* for bodyworkers, nurses and therapists."

Peggy Dawson, director of Service Through Nurturing Touch (NZ)

"*Finding Their Feet* will help parents, carers and early years educators learn more about physical development from pre-birth to two years. As well as learning all about feet, Bernie explores the fascinating aspects of reflexes, sensory integration and movement. There's a mixture of theory and practical ideas and activities presented in an easy to read, relatable style."

Sue Asquith, international early childhood consultant and author (UK)

FINDING THEIR FEET

BERNIE LANDELS

First published 2022 by Bernie Landels

Produced by Indie Experts P/L, Australasia
indieexperts.com.au

Cover design by Daniela Catucci @ Catucci Design
Edited by Anne-Marie Tripp and Samantha Sainsbury
Internal design by Indie Experts
Typeset in 12.25/17 pt Adobe Text Pro by Post Pre-press Group, Brisbane

Unless otherwise noted, illustrations and photos copyright Bernie Landels.

The author would like to thank the following copyright holders, organisations, and individuals for their permission to reproduce copyright images, illustrations, and photos in this book: **1.4:** FCG/Shutterstock.com; **1.5:** Allo4e4ka/Shutterstock.com; **1.6, 5.3:** Xray Computer/Shutterstock.com; **1.9, 3.3, 3.4, 3.5, 3.6, 4.1, 4.2, 5.1, 5.2, 5.4, 5.5, 6.5, 6.6, 7.1, 10.2:** Cynthia Landels; **2.3, 9.1:** Alicia Bennett; **6.7:** Marijs/Shutterstock.com; **7.2:** image and caption republished with permission of John Wiley & Sons, from Whitney G. Cole, Jesse M. Lingeman, and Karen E. Adolph, 'Go Naked: Diapers Affect Infant Walking,' *Developmental Science 6*, no. 15 (November 2012): 783–790, permission conveyed through Copyright Clearance Centre, Inc.; **8.5:** TierneyMJ/Shutterstock.com; **9.2:** You Zhang/Shutterstock.com; **11.1, 11.2, 11.7, 11.11:** Bobux International Ltd/Bobux.co.nz; **11.3:** @Barfussfreaks/Instagram.com; **11.6:** Inch Blue Ltd/InchBlue.com; **11.9:** Softstar Shoes/SoftstarShoes.com; **11.10:** PaperKrane/PaperKrane.com.au; **12.1:** Yok_onepiece/Shutterstock.com; **12.9:** joel bubble ben/Shutterstock.com; **13.1, 13.2:** L. Edgell; **13.3:** K. Bevin.

ISBN 978-0-6452915-0-6 (paperback)
ISBN 978-0-6452915-1-3 (epub)

Disclaimer: The contents of this book are informational only, and not intended to diagnose, treat, cure, or prevent any condition or disease. This book does not substitute professional medical advice or therapeutic evaluation of a child's growth or development. Please consult with your physician or healthcare provider for individually tailored medical advice, diagnoses, or treatment. The author, publishers, and their respective employees and agents are not responsible or liable for any injuries or damage occasioned to any person as a result of reading or following the information contained in this book. References are provided for informational purposes and do not constitute endorsement of any product or service. The use of this book implies your acceptance of this disclaimer.

This book is dedicated to my parents for providing me with a barefoot youth, my sons for teaching me so much about life, and my partner who stands beside me.

CONTENTS

DEAR READER

Thank you for taking the time to read my book; I want to support you and your journey to finding your feet as a parent or carer with a baby who is either waiting to be born or already in your arms.

I truly want you to feel more confident as you navigate your baby's first few years. I may not have all the answers, but I hope this book stimulates you to reach out and explore other avenues of support and help if they are needed, whilst knowing that in your deepened understanding of the human body and in your caring hands, your baby will have the best start at life.

Please use this book as you need – for help and guidance. Dip in and out of it (there's a quick reference guide on page 209), and revisit it with subsequent babies. Write notes in it, use highlighters, fold the corners of particularly helpful pages – then pass it on.

Thank you for welcoming me into your lives.

INTRODUCTION

As a new parent, I had no idea that the foot was an important part of the body, let alone development. There was so much focus on cognitive development alongside standard physical milestones. Being a parent is the most important role I have ever had and I didn't need a degree or masters qualification (though I think even a PhD wouldn't have helped at times!). My two boys were born in 2000 and 2003. At this time, there was the basic information available on breastfeeding, teething, nappy rash, etc. We had no apps or 'Dr Google'. The boys wore hand-me-down clothes and shoes. Much of what I did was based on observations of other parents, advice from family and friends, advertisements and a little bit of intuition or common sense thrown in!

As parents, we want the very best for our children and an important way to do that is by knowing and understanding more about them. The first port of call for information is often the world wide web, and this can provide conflicting information and cause confusion. Many sites will tell you what to do but lacking the 'why'. You are fed information by algorithms largely trying to direct you in a particular way or sell you something.

Advice comes from all sides, with good intention, and we all sieve through it deciding what feels right. We watch others and how they do things; we recall our own experiences, and what our parents did. We trust the experts and what is written as there is just so much to know.

Our external environment, society and marketing are a few factors that influence our decisions with regards to movement and what we wear and products we buy. Many parents feel confused and overloaded by the never-ending pressure and tsunami of information. Parents often only seek help and information when the growth and development of their child falls outside of the normal realm. This means parents are focused on problem-solving after the issue arises rather than preventing the issue from occurring in the first place.

My goal is to inform you of the nuts and bolts of growth and movement, from the feet up, so that you may make more informed decisions and choices. I want you to feel confident trusting your own gut feelings and instincts. After all, who knows your infant better?

This book is all about the importance of your baby 'finding their feet' to set them up developmentally for life. This book will help you make better choices for the young feet in your life. At the same time, you might find it helps you as an adult to move more and live a fuller, healthier life (and keep up with those young feet). This book hopefully also speaks to you as you find your feet as a new parent, second-time-around parent, carer or grandparent.

Babies' feet have never really been written about in any great detail for parents or carers. The upper body, ears, eyes and brain tend to take most of the focus as a baby grows. Breastfeeding, teething and sleeping are common topics amongst parent conversations and forums.

But where do the feet fit in?

Babies use their feet every day from birth. From the age of two, given the opportunity, a child will take 5,000 steps each day on average. By the time they are thirty, they will have taken 51,100,000 steps, which could be as much as 40,000 km (25,000 miles).

Our feet play such an important role in our lives yet from the time we are born, they don't receive the attention they deserve or need.

Milestones are the visual measurements used by most parents to gauge development. Milestones are significant events as the baby moves towards independence. Many parents feel intense pressure for their baby to perform and meet the normal and expected timeframes for milestones such as rolling, crawling and walking. Many parents feel anxious about milestones. Is my baby delayed? Is that normal? Why isn't my baby doing that yet? These are all real concerns and questions throughout the first couple of years.

We hope that our infants will progress through all the milestones in a timely manner, but alas there seems to be more developmental issues seen in children today than in years past. The World Health Organisation met in 2020 to discuss strategies around monitoring and intervention related to child development as their statistics showed 'at least one in six children experience a developmental difficulty.'[1]

I often wonder whether if I had had access to different information when I was a young mum, I would have made different choices for my kids. With more information about early physical development, the how, why and when different things happen as they grow, you can now make more informed decisions.

You can make a difference to your child's future and help them succeed through putting their best foot forward, literally. Taking care of their feet will set up your child for better health in the future – **PREVENTION IS KEY**. There is more at stake than just walking and running. As this book will outline, the feet are the foundation of proper movement and good health throughout the body for life.

Through my work with parents teaching infant massage and ante/postnatal massage, I have witnessed and shared the worry of the mum who has been referred to a physiotherapist for their baby's turning in foot. I've seen a parent's joy of their child's first steps. As a massage and Structural Integration practitioner, I have also seen the result of immobility, poor posture and shoe choice in clients presenting with pain and discomfort.

For you, I have unpacked the research, sifted through the information and applied this to my knowledge of anatomy. I have applied my clinical knowledge and experience, provided the facts, and posed some questions for you all with the aim that you may have more confidence to make the best decisions. I want you to feel confident in the choices you make for your child's health.

This book will take you on a journey from womb to walking. In the coming chapters, you will learn about the body-wide connective tissues; the input and output that happens in response to stimulus; reflexes, receptors and parts of our brain; how and why we move using different theories and ideas; and how the foot is the main source of information on how our body is interacting with the ground. Our feet play an important role in the development of our sense of space and balance in the sensory and perception systems. Without our feet, we have no sense of where we are.

In terms of our overall health, if the feet aren't moving properly, then something else up the chain – ankles or knees – will need to compensate. Good health begins at the feet. What we put on our children's feet – whether we put anything on them at all! – can set up our children for a lifetime of good health. I hope you enjoy our journey together.

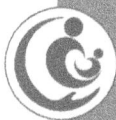

When you see this logo, you'll find activities and ideas for you to use with your baby. Adapt any of these to suit your situation and environment. Be guided by your baby or infant as to how long you do an activity for; their needs come first and we don't want to overstimulate them.

Keep this book handy as a reminder to do something each day.

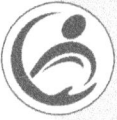

When you see this logo, you'll find experiences for you to do as you read to help your understanding. Consider it research into your own body and capabilities, and permission to move.

Before you turn the page, kick your shoes off. Now we are ready.

CHAPTER 1

FIRST KICKS: THE DEVELOPMENT OF THE FOOT

I CAN STILL REMEMBER BEING KICKED. HOW CAN SUCH A SMALL being take your breath away? I imagined my baby swimming laps, pushing off from each end of the amniotic pool! I since have wondered, what is the significance of those kicks, those pushes, and more importantly, those feet?

Let's take a close-up look at some stages of physical development from the beginning, make some connections and explore what happens before and after those first kicks! Starting at the beginning is important as how humans are formed is the foundation for growth and development; it is where movement starts. Like any journey there is a first step (pardon the pun); let's get your baby's journey to their first steps right.

FROM CONCEPTION

Your baby starts their physical life as a wee cell (zygote). They travel down the fallopian tube to the uterus and snuggle in for the next thirty-five weeks or so before they are ready to venture into the outside world. The journey of life has begun.

From weeks two to eight, your baby is an embryo, a time when all their basic structures are forming.

An embryo grows from the inside out as one self-evolving organism. At the early stages, an embryo transforms into a three-dimensional disc of several folded layers of tissue (IMAGE 1.1). The outer layer is called the ectoderm. The skin, sensory organs, nerves and brain evolve from the ectoderm. The inner layer (endoderm) forms the lining of our gastro-intestinal tube and oesophagus, and is also found in our organs such as the pancreas, liver and thyroid. The folding may explain how at birth tissues that are not connected have similar functions based on their origin.

Between the layers mentioned above, the middle layer (mesoderm) has the cells from which muscles, cartilage, bone and other connective tissues such as blood, fatty tissue and fascia will form.

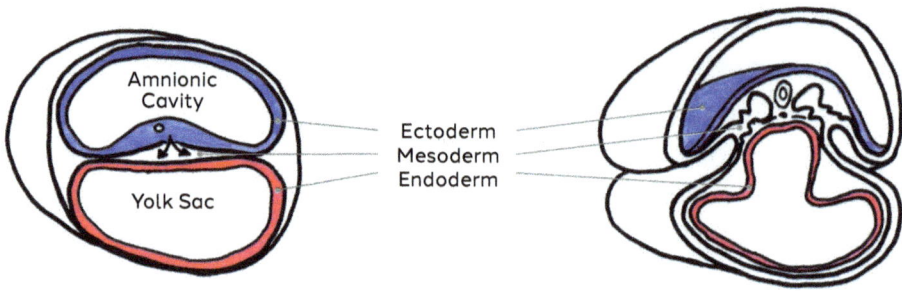

IMAGE 1.1: An embryo is formed from cells gathering together to create different layers, or membranes, as seen on the left. Then embryonic folding occurs (right) to form the different structures such as the gastrointestinal tube from mouth to anus.

Your baby is a 3D living organism from the beginning, evolving from three layers, folding in and around it's heart (IMAGE 1.2). Connected layers, each with a specific purpose and destination, and yet reliant on each other for life.

The human body is very complex, so we are primarily going to focus on the relationship between body (fascia, bones, muscles) and brain (nerves), in relation to physical developmental, milestones and reflexes. Your baby's journey from warm womb to freedom on their two feet.

FASCIA

Fascia is our first stop as it connects everything. It is a thin casing of connective tissue throughout the body. It is everywhere under our skin. Fascia first appears in the middle layer (mesoderm), from around two weeks. As your baby grows, fascia continues to connect, separate and interact with every part of their body.

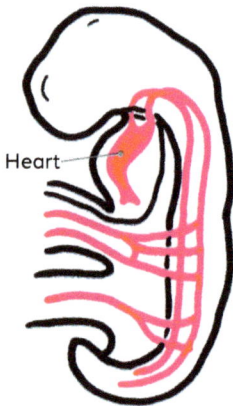

IMAGE 1.2: At four weeks old the embryo's heart begins to beat.

Our fascial system is both fibrous and fluid, forming a gel-like substance that allows for frictionless glide within our body between organs, muscles, bones and nerves. Some fascia is soft and pliable to allow movement and act as a shock absorber. Other fascia, however, is stiff and hard, providing us with stability and support, such as our 'plantar fascia' (you may have heard of the common complaint plantar fasciitis, a painful inflammatory condition of the foot). Fascia adapts to its role and is crucial to our posture and movement.

You may have seen fascia in fresh meat when cooking. If you lift the skin away from a piece of raw chicken meat, the fibrous gooey substance you see is superficial fascia. The white lines inside a beef steak are bands of deeper fascia. Or if you prefer an orange, the pith that surrounds and divides each segment and the covering of each juice vesicle within each segment is like fascia.

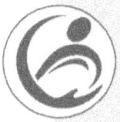

Feel the back of your hand: move your skin over the underlying muscles, tendons, vessels and bones. Hopefully there's lots of glide; this is provided by a superficial layer of fascia just beneath skin.

Fascia is also our richest sensory organ[2] housing millions of nerves, transporting messages to and from the brain to different parts of our body.

So rather than thinking about the body as a bag of individual parts, I believe we need to understand what connects us, the interactions and relationships. Fascia connects everything inside of us and also provides awareness of where we are and how we are moving. I'll explain more as we go.

LIMB BUDS

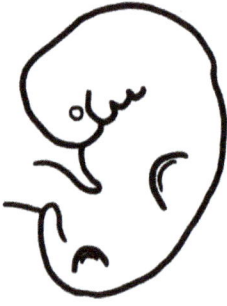

IMAGE 1.3: Limb buds forming on the left (and right) sides of the embryo extend like little paddles.

During their fourth week and at just 4 mm in length, your baby's legs and feet start to grow (IMAGE 1.3). Little bumps called limb buds appear on each side of their lower body. As the buds grow like little paddles, they extend forwards, then rotate inwards; this will allow your baby to eventually stand on two legs. (If they didn't rotate, your baby would have to stay on all fours.) As the limb grows, inside the sea of fascia cells form cartilage structures that will eventually become your baby's bones, while other cells become muscles. Webbed digits separate to give your baby toes and nerve pathways are laid from the brain and spinal cord, exiting at the lower back and tracking down the leg to the toes.

FOOT BONES

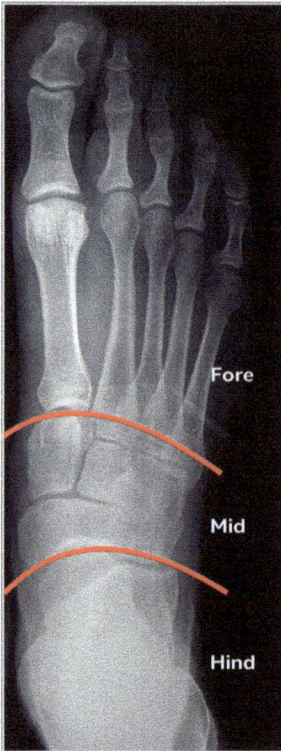

IMAGE 1.4: X-ray image of adult foot bones showing how foot is divided up.

Let's get those kicks really going in the amniotic sea and follow the formation of the foot bones. By week nine, their limb bud looks more like a leg. All structures are in place that will morph into your baby's foot, the bones in the form of cartilage – some of them just tiny dots!

For purposes of describing and understanding movement, the foot is divided up into three parts: fore, mid and hindfoot (IMAGE 1.4).

Ossification (hardening where cartilage becomes bone) starts in the forefoot. The big

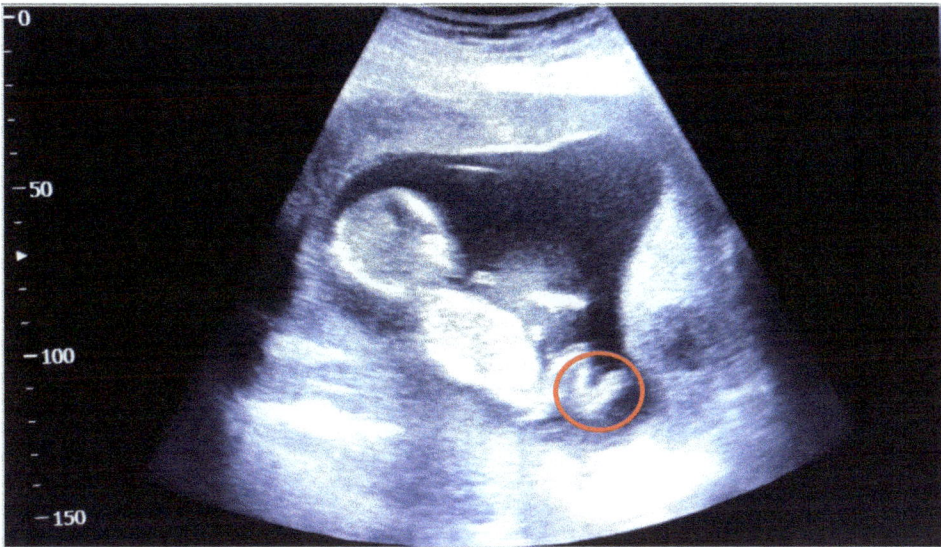

IMAGE 1.5: Ultrasound scan of fetus aged fourteen weeks showing foot.

toe (hallux) and long foot bones (metatarsal rays) lead the way, closely followed by the other toe bones on the tips (distal phalanges). All ten toes can usually be seen at your first anatomy scan at twelve to fourteen weeks (IMAGE 1.5).

Hardening of the bones continues whilst your baby is in the womb with the hindfoot next. The heel bone (calcaneus) becomes visible by the end of the first trimester and the ankle bone (talus) appears shortly after.

The first midfoot bone to grow is the cuboid (square in shape) and it has hardened by birth.

After birth, the final development of what is to be their foundation for posture and movement continues (IMAGE 1.6). By the age of five to six years, your child will have a structure similar to the adult foot, which finally matures in their late teens. That's right, foot bones take their time to develop.

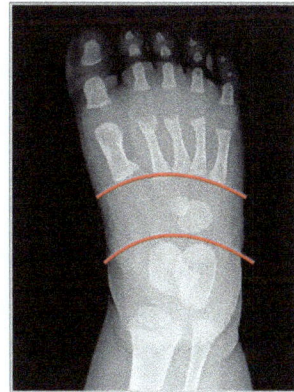

IMAGE 1.6: X-ray image of six-month-old infant's foot. Divisions of hind, mid and forefoot also shown. Notice the lack of midfoot bones.

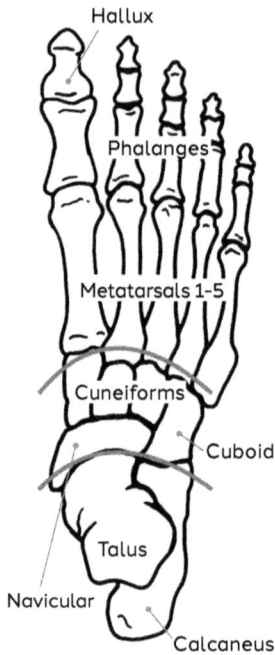

Hallux

Phalanges

Metatarsals 1-5

Cuneiforms

Cuboid

Talus

Navicular

Calcaneus

IMAGE 1.7: Adult foot structure looking down showing the unique shapes of the bones.

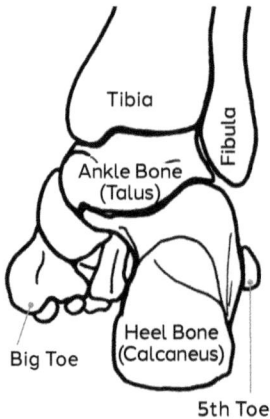

Tibia

Fibula

Ankle Bone (Talus)

Heel Bone (Calcaneus)

Big Toe

5th Toe

IMAGE 1.8: Adult right foot structure from behind. Notice how the heel bone is positioned more on the outside of the foot.

Look down at your feet. You have twenty-six bones in each foot; that's nearly a quarter of all your bones (52 out of 206) in your feet! Your baby will start with around 300 bones compared to your 206; theirs are mostly flexible cartilage as ossification and fusing will happen over time.

If you were to look closely at the bones of your feet (IMAGE 1.7), you would notice they each have a unique shape. From behind (IMAGE 1.8), you will notice the heel bone is NOT under the middle of the lower leg bones. The ankle bone (talus) is nestled between the heel bone and the lower leg bones (tibia and fibula). 'Talus' is also the name given to a large, loose stone on the side of a mountain so you could think of the heel bone (calcaneus) being the mountain. It is after all the largest foot bone. The ankle bone that sits on top has NO muscles/tendons attaching to it (loose stone on side of mountain). Stability is provided by ligaments and movement generated from and influenced by its position between the heel bone and lower leg bones. The ankle bone therefore plays a key role in connecting the leg to the foot and in movement.

The developed midfoot, in addition to the cuboid, has three small wedge-like bones called cuneiforms (*cuneius* is Latin for 'wedge'). These bones are narrower on the bottom, creating a bridge-like formation. Between these three bones and the ankle bone is our navicular, named for its boat shape. It's something of a stretch to one's imagination, but I like to think of it as a boat riding the movement of the ankle bone and the navigator guiding the cuneiforms.

The arrangement of our uniquely-shaped bones, suspended, floating inside, allows for both support and mobility. The squarer, more solid hind/midfoot bones can withstand impact forces. The longer forefoot bones allow for movement and provide leverage, like the long lever of a catapult. The smaller toe bones are designed for balance and stability. Connective tissue keeps the bones apart and with the support of ligaments and muscles arches are formed.

ARCHES

Baby feet often appear flat. The absence of arches is a transitional phase in development.[3] A healthy adult foot has three arches: a medial (inside) longitudinal arch, which is the most commonly known one that goes from the front of the heel to the ball of the big toe; a lateral (outside) longitudinal arch that goes from the heel bone to the start of the little toe; and a long transverse (across) arch running the length of the foot from in front of the heel bone to the ends of the five metatarsals (toe bones). Together they create a dome-like shape under your foot which, when loaded, provides support along with the potential for more dynamic movement.

The reason your baby's feet look flat (IMAGE 1.9) is because of fat pads on their soles that appear in utero. These should disappear by the time your child is five. If you think back to the formation of the bones, this fat pad fills the space of the inner arch where the midfoot bones are slow to develop. They serve to protect the young, underdeveloped feet from overloading when your baby starts standing

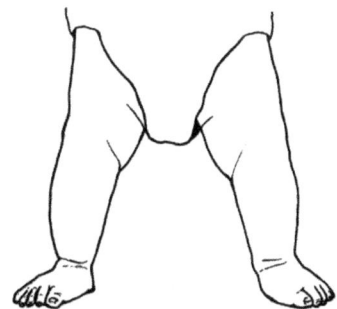

IMAGE 1.9: Baby feet often appear flat, to protect and increase sensory awareness.

and walking. I also believe that the fat pad increases the surface area of the foot and as it is full of sensory receptors, it increases the information that can be taken in.

With the toe bones and heel developing early we see the foundation forming. As the foot matures, ligaments, muscles and fascia support the uniquely-shaped bones to form the dome-shaped arches. These bones create a tripod of support, between the heel and the bases of the big and little toes (IMAGE 1.10).

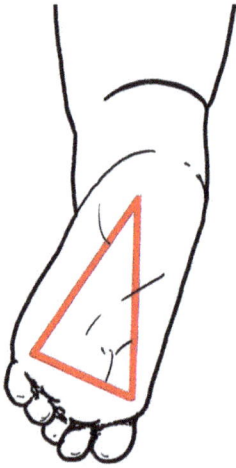

IMAGE 1.10: Infant foot showing tripod of support from heel to ends of first and fifth metatarsal bones.

How many times have you been out for a meal and sat at a table that's wobbly? Guaranteed that table had four legs but was only using three! A tripod, three points of contact, is a stable structure. When we stand, our weight is distributed to the base of our tripods in each foot. This base should allow us to stand and balance on one leg. We will bring the tripods and arches alive when we look at walking, as they both have a crucial part to play when we move.

MUSCLES

The last part of our anatomy 101 lesson (for now) deals with muscles.

As your baby's limb buds grow outwards, cells from the middle layer form muscle fibres. Bundles of these become individual muscles. Your baby will start using these muscles and practicing movement in the womb. Like learning anything new, they will be quite uncoordinated to begin with! This all contributes to forming neural connections, learning and laying down movement pathways.

Remember how fascia is everywhere? It surrounds each muscle fibre and muscle, even groups of muscles. It's like fascia has pockets that muscle cells fill – are we one big muscle separated and connected by fascia?

Fascia provides glide between muscles and groups of muscles, and helps increase muscle power. The containment of the muscles increases the pressure inside the wrapping and the added stiffness (remember how fascia can be both fluid and fibrous) helps the muscles produce more force.

Back down at the foot, there are nineteen small muscles in each foot. The arrangement of four layers and nine compartments provides both strength and mobility. Over thirty ligaments support each foot and ankle. Ten larger muscles that originate in the lower leg compartments also assist to stabilise, support and move our ankles, feet and toes. Most of the lower leg muscles are tendon by the time they reach the foot. A tendon is a thickening of connective tissue, a bit like rope, that emerges from the muscle to attach to the bone.

The Achilles tendon is probably one you are familiar with; it's the largest tendon and connects the calf muscles (gastrocnemius/soleus) to the heel bone (calcaneus). Connecting the heel bone with the toes is the plantar fascia that is a thickening to provide resistance and support.

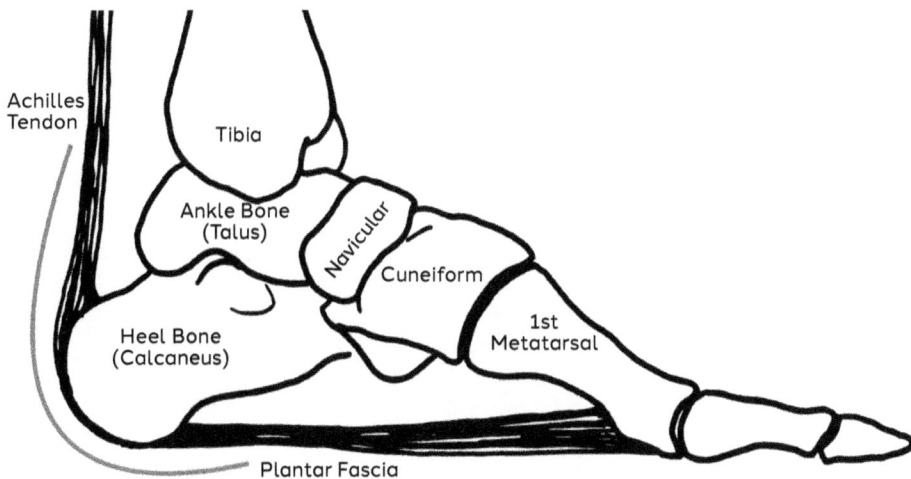

IMAGE 1.11: Side view of adult foot showing the Achilles tendon and plantar fascia connecting by a layer of fascial tissue around the heel bone.

The Achilles tendon and plantar fascia are connected fascially around the heel (IMAGE 1.11).

Locations of regular high impact or strain are reinforced by laying more fascia down. This explains the plantar fascia on the sole of the foot. Laying down these reinforcements happens over time with the development and practice of natural movement.

For such a small part of the body there is a lot down there – nerves, blood vessels, muscles, bone and more – all originating from the outer and middle layers (ectoderm and mesoderm) of the embryo coming together to form your baby's cute little foot.

TOENAILS

Let's finish this chapter at the toes. Have you ever wondered why we have toenails?

The front and back of each limb bud has a ridge of tissue from the outer layer (ectoderm) that becomes the nails on the tips of the toes.

The nails are composed of layers of dead, compacted cells which is why it doesn't hurt to cut them.

Can you imagine life without nails? We all know how useful fingernails are. The primary purpose of nails is protection. They also provide resistance or counter pressure which in turn increases sensitivity and helps with balance.

Have you ever stubbed your toe? If it wasn't for your toenail, I assure you it would have hurt much more.

HERE'S SOMETHING TO THINK ABOUT

Fingers have fingertips, but toes don't have toetips …
Yes, you can tiptoe but not tipfinger!

CHAPTER 2

FEELING THEIR FEET: SENSORY DEVELOPMENT

SENSORY START

Inside the safety of the womb, growing day by day, your baby is taking on the form that we recognise to be human. By week twelve, your baby's sensory organs (ears and nose) have fully developed from thickenings of the outer layer of ectoderm. You start to feel your baby's movements (called 'quickening') during the second trimester.

Your baby's sensory system relating to touch is developing from around the time that the first kick is felt and continues developing after birth. Inside their body are a range of sensory receptors for providing information to the brain, different receptors for different sensations. You could liken a receptor to a language translator: they receive one language (stimuli) in and translate it to another language for someone else (the brain) to understand.

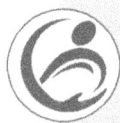

> Wiggle your toes and think about the temperature of your feet and how they feel. Your feet just had a two-way conversation with different parts of your brain.

In your conversation, sensory receptors in the feet that feel pressure (mechanoreceptors), pain (nociceptors) and temperature (thermo-receptors) sent messages to your sensory brain about how they, your feet, are doing way down there. At the same time, your motor brain relays messages to your feet to wiggle your toes to increase the sensation and thus the connection. The motor part of your brain engaged your proprioceptors in the conversation by letting you know where your feet were and what they were doing.

HOMUNCULUS – BODY-BRAIN CONNECTION

When on holiday with my family, we visited the Ottobock Science Centre in Berlin, Germany, where they develop prosthetic limbs. It was there that I first met 'Homunculus'. He is a very small humanoid/human-like creature. (Yes, he is male, but equally could be female, of course!) (IMAGE 2.1)

Homunculus is a visual model that helps us understand the sensing and moving body. It is a 'map' of the somatosensory (somatic means physical human body) and motor systems in the brain.[4] The bigger the body part on Homunculus, the more sensitive or more capable of fine movement it is. Check out the

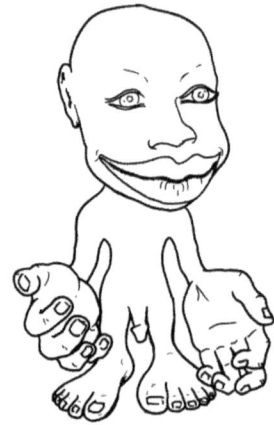

IMAGE 2.1: Homunculus – the bigger the body part, the more sensitive or capable of fine motor skills.

hands, feet and lips. If you think about your own body and your senses, these are related to the most 'sensory' parts of your body. With movement, the finer the motor control required, the larger the area mapped in our brain. For example, the area responsible for the dexterity of our hand is much larger than the area dedicated to the thigh.

I feel the feet are a forgotten sensory and motor organ so I have given them an upgrade and made them bigger. Hopefully by the end of this book you'll agree 'he' needs bigger feet!

BRAINY BITS

Let's have a quick anatomy lesson of our brain.

When I think of the brain, I think of a walnut, though the brain is much more moist! The walnut grows from a stem on a branch, in the same way our brain grows from the brain stem. The brain stem is the first part of the brain to develop and controls autonomic functions such as heartbeat.

Crack open a walnut and you will find it is divided into two halves, each of which has a wrinkled outer surface. In the brain, the two halves (hemispheres) are connected by the corpus callosum, a bundle of over 200 million nerve fibres that send messages back and forth. Both sides of the brain are covered by a thin layer of grey tissue that contains most of the brain cells. This is where the information comes in from our senses: touch, taste, smell, sight and sound.

Each side of the brain is divided into four sections, or lobes. The frontal, parietal and occipital lobes are arranged from the front across the top to the back, like a mohawk. The temporal lobes sit either side (like the shaved hair around the ears).

Homunculus's sensory map (IMAGE 2.2) is located in the parietal lobe, both left and right, and receives input such as touch, pain and

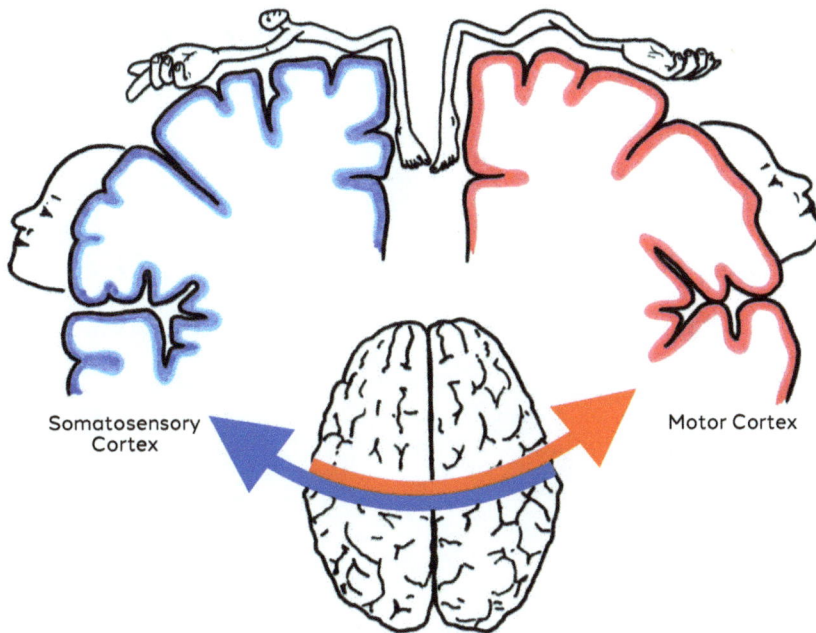

Somatosensory Cortex

Motor Cortex

IMAGE 2.2: Homunculus sensory and motor maps in the brain.

temperature from sensory receptors throughout the body. The larger parts of the Homunculus body have more, densely packed receptors and so claim a greater proportion of the brain.

Homunculus's motor map (SEE IMAGE 2.2) is found across the frontal lobe (left and right) and sends messages to receptors for controlling movement of different parts of the body.

Hidden under the front part of our brain, there is a special part of the brain called the insular cortex, whose key function is the perception of the state of our body and how we feel, such as warm, hungry, thirsty, sore, sick, even itchy. This internal awareness, or interoception, is key for our survival, and the feet play a vital role in providing input.

There are of course other parts of the brain involved with balance, coordination, motor control, how we move and sense the world. What is important to know is that the brain and body together have continuous feedback loops allowing us to stand, walk, dance and respond to our internal and external environments.

We are born with 100–200 billion nerve cells. That's 250–500 thousand growing each minute during pregnancy![5] At birth, these nerve cells are ready to connect and transmit, and the first two years are critical for the successful development of these neural pathways.

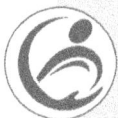

HERE'S A LITTLE FUN TEST FOR YOU

Take two pins or toothpicks, even the nibs of two pens – anything with a small, pointed tip.

Holding the pins about 10 mm apart, and without looking, touch one of your fingertips lightly with the tips of both pins at the same time. Try touching different fingers – what do you feel? Repeat on your toe pads – what's the most sensitive region for you?

Hopefully you found that on the smaller areas/body parts you could feel two tips. This is due to the tips touching different receptor fields and the nervous system sending two messages to the brain (as more sensory receptors are located in a small area). On the larger body parts, it probably felt like only one tip, as a larger area has fewer receptors and both tips would have been landing in the same receptor field.

Whilst there is some debate about the accuracy of the 'Homunculus' neurological map, I'd like you to keep the Homunculus image of big feet in your mind as you read this book. Remember all that practice and searching for sensory input your baby performs whilst in the womb? The feet are a sensory rich part of the body hungry for stimulus and ready for action, so don't hide them away! (IMAGE 2.3)

We have 250 million sensory receptors in our fascia,[6] which is three times more than motor receptors. And we have more sensory receptors

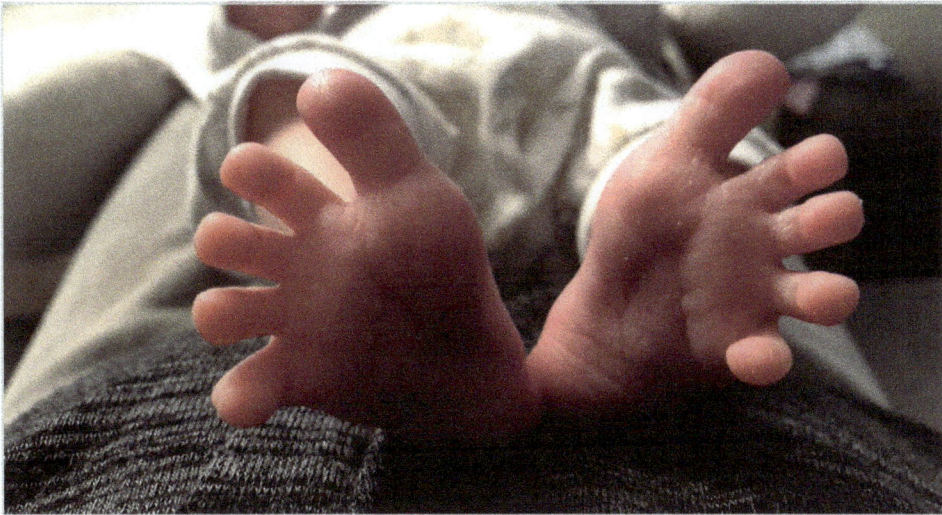

IMAGE 2.3: Evy (aged one month) reaching out to touch the world. (Photo: A Bennett)

in our feet than anywhere else in our body. Information received by the sensory receptors is rapidly communicated to the brain, through nerves that are within our body's fascial fabric.

No wonder when we walk barefoot on gravel it hurts so much, as the sharp edges of small stones touch each and every small receptor field. If our brain is not used to such stimulation, it will sense it as dangerous, similar to walking on hot sand or the hot tarmac at the beach car park. What comes next is the awkward *oo-ee-oo-aa* dance as we try not to put our feet down (less foot-to-ground contact means less receptor contact) and scramble to our towel or race to the car! The sensation we feel, however, occurs in the brain, not our feet. Our brain is just unaccustomed to such extreme sensations, so it automatically sends messages of danger. The pain response is the brain's way of protecting us from tissue damage when interpreting a sensation as potentially dangerous; this drives a reaction, in this instance withdrawal and speed.

The more your baby experiences different surfaces such as carpet, grass, sand, dirt, mud, or water in the first few months and years, the more informed their brain will be, the more familiar the sensations will be and hopefully the less their pain response. Note: we are not trying to achieve any super-human feats here like walking on hot coals, just experiences in our everyday environments.

I recall the day I took my son Nick to the beach for the first time. He wasn't yet walking so I plonked him down to sit on the sand without a thought of what it would be like for him. Barefooted, the ground moved as he kicked, gave way and moulded with his body. The sand was fine enough for him to pick up a handful only to watch it trickle through his fingers. I wish I could have captured that moment and known what was going through his mind ...

TOUCH

Touch is the first of the five senses to develop with receptors everywhere in your baby's body – except for their head. This is probably good given their poor head is likely to be fairly squished and battered as it makes its way down through the birth canal, all going well, leading your baby out into the world. This is also why the midwife and birthing assistants guiding your baby's arrival can attach monitors or suction cups and use forceps to help delivery.

Now back to those kicks, and probably a few punches have started too! According to scientists at the University College of London, spontaneous movements of the hands and feet are the start of making important brain–body connections and help your baby negotiate the outside world – no more womb-service![7] The researchers measured brainwaves in newborns and found that movement of the right hand generated brainwaves in the left hemisphere of the brain and vice versa. With a similar neural connection of the feet to the spine, stimulation and movement of the right foot would also generate brainwaves in the left brain. The research suggests that reaching and kicking out helps develop the sensory input region of the brain and initiates the communication between the two hemispheres, and is how an infant begins to get a sense of their own body.

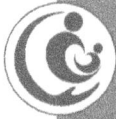

HOW TO INCREASE YOUR BABY'S SENSORY INPUT AT THE FEET

As newborns

- Massaging and holding their wee feet not only provides them stimulation, touch is a great way to connect with your baby.
- Blow on their feet so they can feel the gentle breeze and warmth of your breath.
- At bath time just dip their feet in first, letting them feel water on their feet rather than starting with full body immersion.
- Place your baby at the bottom of their bassinet/cot so they can touch the walls with the sole of their foot.

As they get older

- When your baby is lying on their back, place different soft/textured objects at their feet for them to feel, even newspaper/cellophane that they can scrunch with their toes.
- Vary the surfaces they lie/move on. Encourage your child to explore the outdoors more so they can experience grass, dirt, sand and gravel.
- Here's a sensory game to play together: lay out different containers with contents such as jelly, warm water, and cooked spaghetti. Let your child feel the different sensations, then with their eyes shut or a blindfold on, can your child, using only their feet, guess what the items are?
- Lay out a sensory trail for your child to walk on, using dried leaves, sand, grass, dirt, carpet, paper, etc.
- Create a barefoot-friendly home.

THE LEARNING BRAIN

From birth throughout life, the brain and body are learning together, with the foundations begin being laid in the womb. The brain stem kicks off with involuntary movements known as primitive reflexes. From here your baby will work on building strong postural and movement patterns, and develop their perception and self-awareness – all needed before development of language, understanding and learning can occur (IMAGE 2.4).

Are you ready to help your baby grow and develop great foundations?

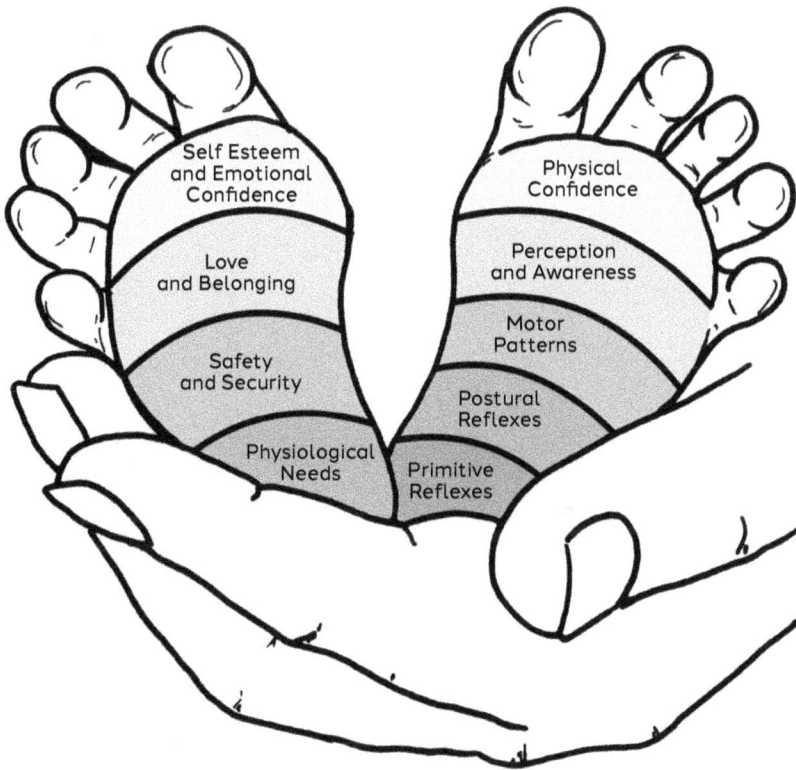

IMAGE 2.4: Foundations of basic needs (left) alongside basic movement progression (right), both are required for your baby to build confidence and a sense of self. These foundations will then support the development of fine motor skills, language, understanding and thinking. Gaps or weaknesses may hinder your child's development and chance to jump into this world grounded and well balanced on both feet.

CHAPTER 3

FIRST MOVEMENTS: REFLEXES

I HAD NEVER HELD A NEWBORN BEFORE NICK ARRIVED IN MY arms. In front of me was this bundle of cuteness overflowing with potential but unable to move very far by himself ... yet!

REFLEXES

The first movements of your newborn baby are primitive reflexes, designed for survival and a blueprint for body-brain development. They are innate, unconscious and unlearned responses that in time, with normal development and maturity of the central nervous system, are replaced with postural reflexes, voluntary behaviours and motor skills.[8] Primitive reflexes appear in sequence (see chart on page 189) and are considered to be integrated when your baby does not automatically respond to a certain stimulus and has control over what they do.

Reflexes are a significant part of your baby's developmental milestones, their first teacher of movement patterns that will help them learn to roll, crawl and walk. These repeated automatic movements develop the brain, especially the frontal lobe where the 'Homunculus' motor map is, each new movement pattern building new neural pathways and connections.

You may be familiar with the grasp reflex of the hands, allowing your baby to hold your finger or grab your hair. In infant massage classes when we do face massage, I'm often asked, 'Why does she stick out her tongue when I rub her cheeks?' That's the rooting reflex. In addition to the sucking reflex, these are all survival reflexes. There is the startle reflex, also called the Moro reflex, which is an example of a motor reflex where a change in position or a loud sound evokes a physical response in the body. It's this reflex that triggers your baby's first breath.

Reflexes are part of newborn screening tests, assessed by moving the baby's head, and stroking its foot, cheek, spine and hand. Reflexes are also used to examine for neurological conditions such as cerebral palsy. More recently it has been found that retained reflexes may lead to other developmental delays. The Millennium Cohort Study[9] started tracking nearly 20,000 children born in the United Kingdom between 2000 and 2002. This study found that those infants with delayed neuro-motor development in their first year presented with reduced cognitive development and behavioural issues at the age of five. A more recent, smaller study[10] of four- to five-year-olds found an increasing number were starting school with retained reflexes and without the physical skills necessary to support their education and learning.

The integration of primitive reflexes can be interrupted by:

Pre-birth
- exposure to drugs
- poor nutrition
- emotional stress.

Birthing
- caesarean section
- premature birth
- instrument-assisted birth
- long or complicated labour.

Post-birth
- excessive swaddling
- minimal floor and tummy time
- overuse of carriers, walkers, car seats
- overuse of external stimulation (TV/mobile devices) resulting in no movement.

As a child grows, if any reflex is retained (not integrated) they may struggle with social skills, problem-solving, or focusing, and present symptoms such as:

- reduced or increased muscle tone
- hypersensitivity
- anxiety
- clumsiness
- poor hand-eye coordination
- motion sickness
- bed-wetting beyond five years
- speech challenges
- toe-walking.

It is important to know that what you are seeing when your baby moves or reacts in a certain way may be a reflex, and it is a stage they should transition through. Reflexes are important in the development of the central nervous system. It is also important to know what they are for and when they should integrate. Just like when building a house it's easier to lay the wiring in the early stages, **YOU CAN HELP YOUR CHILD BUILD SOLID FOUNDATIONS WITH GOOD WIRING OF THEIR REFLEXES.**

Ahead we will explore a few of the reflexes relating to the feet, balance and movement. Reflexes are crucial for the developmental milestones of rolling, crawling and walking.

Plantar reflex

If you stroke or press the sole of your baby's foot, they will curl their toes. In other words, the receptors on their sole sent a message via the pressure receptors along the spinal cord to the brain causing the toes to flex. The plantar reflex develops in the womb at around eleven weeks. Whilst it is similar to the grasp reflex in the hand, the plantar reflex is weaker. This could be due to the fat pad on the foot or shortness of your baby's cute toes. (Humans don't use toes like our monkey cousins to climb and hold.) Integration of this reflex allows the toes to lie flat and be lifted, both required for standing and walking **(IMAGE 3.1).**

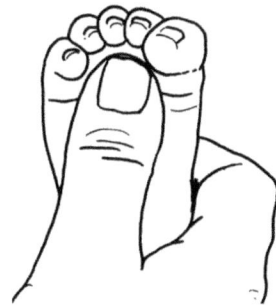

IMAGE 3.1: Plantar reflex: toes curl in response to pressure.

Babinski reflex

The Babinski sign or reflex in the foot is stimulated by stroking the outside of the sole from the heel to and along under the toes to the big toe (in a 'L' shape). It will result in your baby's big toe lifting with or without the toes spreading (IMAGE 3.2).

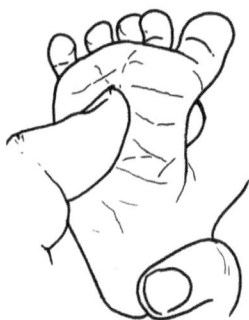

IMAGE 3.2: Babinski reflex: toes lift and spread when foot stroked.

You may notice that the plantar and Babinski reflexes are opposite in action, both serving to provide support and balance, and movement respectively. They prepare the feet for walking.

Think about how far the toes are from the brain for a moment. Curling and uncurling the toes is the brain exercising its longest motor pathway and feedback loop, from the motor cortex to the tips of the toes and back (right brain to left toes and vice versa).

Retained plantar or Babinski reflexes may present as:

- delayed walking
- poor balance and eye-foot coordination
- toe-walking
- difficulty wearing shoes.

Allowing the toes and feet to be free, experiencing different stimuli as they grow, and infant massage may help with integrating these two reflexes.

Stepping reflex

The stepping reflex develops perhaps as part of the sensory mapping process in the womb or as part of building the neural pathways for walking. The reflex is observed after birth when you hold your baby with their feet touching your lap or other surface, and they look like they are walking or want to jump. Their bodies are not yet strong enough to walk – and as we will see they have a lot more learning to do before they walk – but this reflex shows that the baby's brain is already preparing for their future.

Your baby's feet are connected not only to their legs but all the way up to their head so let's look at some other reflexes that are important to balance and moving.

Asymmetrical tonic neck reflex (ATNR)

This reflex develops in utero, around the time that you feel the baby's first movements. When your baby turns their head, their arm and leg on the same side extend – and there's that kick (IMAGE 3.3). ATNR assists your baby to move in the womb and helps in the birthing process. During 'normal' vaginal delivery, the newborn has to turn 180 degrees and this asymmetrical movement helps with rotating down the birth canal, a bit like a corkscrew.[11] This reflex can also help babies to free their airway when on their tummy, assist with rolling, help develop a sense of each side of their body and is part of the hand-eye coordination training. ATNR is integrated with the development of motor skills in the first six to nine months. You will see your baby turning their head to look at different things without either arm extending or moving away from their body and bringing their hand towards their face.

Retained ATNR has been associated with poor hand-eye coordination leading to poor fine motor skills (e.g., writing), and difficulty with activities requiring the arm or leg crossing the midline of the body.

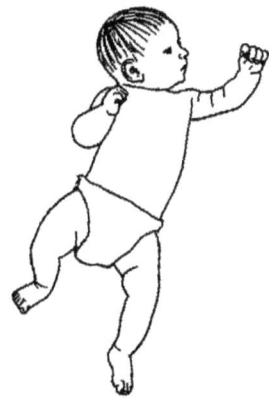

IMAGE 3.3: Asymmetrical tonic neck reflex: arm and leg extend when they turn their head to that side.

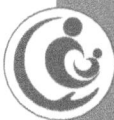

Bauer crawling reflex

Developing in utero around the twenty-eight-week mark, this reflex is another contributor to all those kicks. Similar to the stepping reflex, when pressure is applied to the soles of the baby's feet, but this time when the baby is lying on their stomach, a crawling or creeping response occurs. Also assisting in the mapping of 'Homunculus' and the birthing process, this reflex remains for around three months, making way for another crawling reflex to start emerging.

Symmetrical tonic neck reflex (STNR)

STNR, sometimes referred to as a 'crawling reflex', is present at birth for a few days. It is a survival reflex assisting the newborn to crawl up the belly[12] to find the nipple in the same way blind puppies and kittens do. It then disappears and reappears anywhere from four to nine months of age to help with preparation for crawling. The wide timeframe is perhaps a reflection of experience and opportunity, for example with more time spent on their tummy the baby may develop this reflex earlier.

STNR helps get your baby up on their hands and knees and then learn to use the lower and upper parts of the body independently of each other. At first you may observe your baby rocking back and forth when on hands and knees. Their head drives this movement, as they look up their arms will straighten, knees and hips bend behind, the opposite happening when they look down. Using both of their arms and their legs together will also help integrate ATNR and eventually get them up standing. STNR is integrated with success in moving their head independently of their body, at around six to nine months (IMAGE 3.4).

Similar to ATNR, a child with a retained integrating STNR may present with poor hand-eye coordination. They may prefer to scoot on their bottom or bear crawl on hands and feet, slouch and be clumsy.

Tummy time is important preparation for integrating STNR. As your baby develops strength and control of their head, they are able

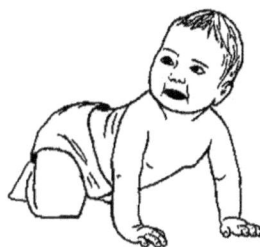

IMAGE 3.4: Integration of the STNR allows for independent head movement.

to practice the different ways to move. They may push up their shoulders, lift their tummy off the ground, push their upper body back or pull their knees up under their hips, eventually managing to coordinate both together with the occasional faceplant.

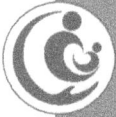

ACTIVITIES TO HELP YOUR BABY AND THEIR STNR

- Keep your baby's knees and feet free so they can sense the floor.
- Place objects or provide motivation for them to look up, which drives the head end.
- Allow your baby time to rock back and forth without being in a hurry to encourage crawling.
- Get down and rock back and forth with them.

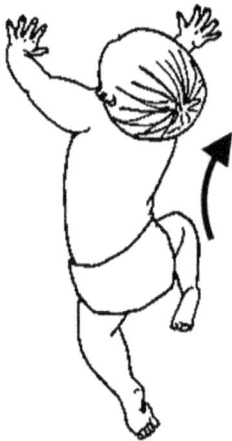

IMAGE 3.5: Spinal Galant: baby side bends in response to being stroked next to their spine.

Spinal Galant reflex

Another reflex emerging in utero, like the ATNR, this reflex has asymmetrical movements that help your baby travel down the birth canal. The spinal Galant (IMAGE 3.5) reflex generates a side flexion of the body when the baby is stimulated on either side of the spine. This reflex is important for getting the hips moving as they do in crawling and walking and should be integrated within six to nine months.

This reflex has a close link to the inner ear and balance (vestibular system). Signs such as poor concentration and posture may be present, along with fidgeting, problems rolling and – believe it or not – bedwetting, may present if not integrated fully.

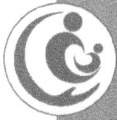

ACTIVITIES TO HELP INTEGRATE THE SPINAL GALANT REFLEX

- Carry and rock your baby in your arms.
- Give your baby a back massage during tummy time.
- When your baby is lying on their back, hold their legs and gently rock them so their head nods up and down.

Landau reflex

With developing muscle tone and strength in your baby's spine, the Landau reflex (IMAGE 3.6) appears, allowing your baby to lift their head and chest, freeing their arms and hands to reach for toys and objects. You will notice their legs will also start lifting. Observed from around three months, this reflex may last up to three years.

Spending time on their tummy again is important. Place objects nearby and encourage family members to get down low to motivate your baby to lift their head and reach out with their hands.

Poor motor development and being clumsy may be signs this reflex has not fully integrated.

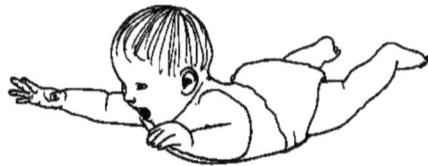

IMAGE 3.6: Landau: head, chest, arms and legs able to lift and extend simultaneously.

> When my boys were little, I recall lying on my back and balancing them on my lower legs so they felt like they were flying. At first, I'd hold their hands but as they grew in confidence they would let go – they loved it, and little did I know that I was helping integrate their Landau reflex!

There are also two reflexes associated with the vestibular system – the inner ear tonic labyrinthine reflex (TLR) and the vestibulo-ocular reflex (VOR). These two reflexes assist your child with navigating the first three to four years, and beyond.

Tonic labyrinthine reflex (TLR)

The tonic labyrinthine reflex (TLR) has two whole-body responses, each triggered by the flexion or extension of the baby's neck. The forward response occurs when the baby looks down (neck flexion), and their arms and legs all flex or curl forwards into the body too, like in the fetal position. The backwards response occurs when the baby looks upwards (neck extension), and their arms and legs extend out and straighten, a little like the Landau reflex.

The TLR forward response emerges in utero around twelve weeks, with the TLR backward response not emerging until after birth. I do wonder if during a natural vaginal delivery, as the baby travels down the birth canal, head extending to negotiate the passage through the mother's pelvis, that last push is created by the baby straightening their legs. I'm not sure where the arms extending or straightening may fit into my theory, though my younger son, Ben, was born in a Superman pose with one arm up leading the way!

Even though the TLR backward response looks similar to the Landau and Moro reflexes, the TLR is related to the inner ear, hence driven by a change in the baby's head position. The labyrinth is part of the inner ear complex, and is responsible for balance.

Flexion and extension change and develop the muscle tone of the back and front of the body, with both responses playing a key role in helping your baby adapt and respond to the new forces they experience in gravity. It is therefore important that your baby has the opportunity to develop both responses equally, as integration of the TLR is critical for developing independent head control, muscle tone, balance and proprioception. The TLR is therefore, like other reflexes, training for crawling, standing and walking.

The forward TLR integrates around three to four months of age, with the backwards TLR integrating from three to nine months, though may linger throughout the child's first two or three years.

Given that the TLR is one of opposite actions (flexion/extension), it makes sense that if the forward or backward response is retained, you would see two different scenarios. A child with a retained forward TLR will present with hypotonicity (weak muscle tone), and may also present symptoms such as:

- tilting their head to one side, or leaning their head on hand/arm
- hunched posture
- difficulty lifting arms overhead when dressing themselves or climbing
- difficulty going downstairs
- a 'W' sitting position as they seek more support.

A retained forward response may be responsible for hyper-mobility in some people, as well.

A child with a retained backward TLR, however, will present with hypertonicity, also known as 'stiff baby syndrome'. Tension in the lower neck and shoulders may also be observed, as the child may opt to use these parts of their body to achieve head control rather than the higher neck vertebrae (C1-3). Their overall balance will be poor, with associated motion sickness, vertigo and a possible fear of heights.

Hypertonicity may be a result of birth trauma or medical procedures, and what comes to mind for me is the Moro reflex, which triggers when a baby is suddenly startled by a loud noise or sudden movement. Staying in an extended or stiff position, as in the Moro reflex reaction, may limit the integration of the backward TLR response. If this response is still active it may lead to:

- toe-walking
- difficulty walking upstairs
- spatial challenges
- challenges with crossing the midline, affecting crawling and walking.

The TLR really is a reflex about balance – balance both in terms of your baby in the world and in terms of integrating. Try to limit the time they spend in car seats and buggies, or propped up in seats, all of which keep them in the flexed position.

Activities on the floor, with the baby on their front and back, will give your baby the opportunity to develop and integrate their TLR. It is completely normal to see your baby arch their back when lying on their back, almost balancing on their head and legs, and it may look like they are trying to roll. I believe the TLR, and its integration, contributes to the successful development of rolling – more on that later.

All these reflexes contribute to the development of balance and movement, preparing your baby for life in the upright world. Some also contribute to successful visual and auditory processing. While all primitive reflexes should integrate over time and transition into different postural reflexes, there is one reflex that remains throughout our lives. Let's take a moment to explore this special reflex.

Vestibulo-ocular reflex (VOR)

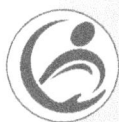

Take a moment and while you keep reading, tilt your head to the left, then to the right. Did you notice that you were able to stay focused on the words (hopefully without feeling queasy)?

Stability of vision, even when your head is moving, is achieved through the development of the VOR. Messages were sent to your brain that your head was moving and your brain adjusted the muscles of your eyes so you could keep reading. This is an important reflex for babies to develop when they start to move more and eventually walk.

The inner ear and parts of the brain responsible for sensory information related to balance and eye movements make up the vestibular system. This system, along with proprioception, uses a continual feedback loop to process information from inside into actions. This information is essential for coordination, balance and control of movement. For example, as your baby starts moving, proprioceptors tell them where their head is, where their right foot is, their foot's relationship to their mouth, and how much effort is needed to get it into their mouth.

All the movement your baby experienced and practiced in the womb provided the brain with information and helped start development of these two internal sensory systems, along with the sensory and motor maps depicted by Homunculus.

After birth, your baby will need further development of the interconnections between the brain and their vestibular system to help them become upright and able to function in gravity. Being carried in your arms or a sling, moved, massaged and played with are some of the best ways to further stimulate and strengthen these balance systems. In fact, any kind of movement in many directions can be perfect: swinging, spinning and rocking all help.

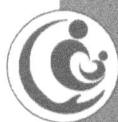

ACTIVITIES TO HELP STIMULATE YOUR BABY'S VESTIBULAR SYSTEM

Early months

- Hold your baby securely under their armpits and support their head as you lift them up and down, varying speed and height (keeping their safety in mind).
- Cradle them in your arms and turn around in a circle (don't get too dizzy yourself!).
- Sit with them in a rocking chair or on an exercise ball – rocking or bouncing.
- Hold them securely on your knee and bounce them, swaying them forward and back, left and right.

WARNING: DOING ANY OF THESE MOVEMENTS STRAIGHT AFTER A FEED MAY HAVE AN UNDESIRABLE OUTCOME.

Once head control established

- Hold your baby under their armpits and 'fly' them around the room as you slowly spin.
- Lie on the floor, bend your knees and place your baby facedown on your lower legs and then move your legs around (also a great workout for you!).
- Tummy time, with your infant pushing and propping themselves up on their elbows. Incorporate looking at books. Join them lying on the floor.

Once crawling and walking

- Encourage backward motion as this will enhance their proprioception as they will use their eyes to guide movement less.
- Crawling and walking up and down slopes.
- Slides and swings at the park.
- Walk the plank – place a long piece of wood 3"/8 cm wide securely on a flat surface and help your toddler crawl or walk along it, both forward and backward.
- Floor swimming – with your infant lying on their tummy have them do a breast stroke action with their arms to lift their torso off the floor.
- Somersaults on the floor are a great activity. Help them get started and guide them. When was the last time you did a forward roll?

Reflexes are key to development and your baby needs a variety of positions and stimulation to help integrate them. Any retained reflexes may affect your infant's behaviour. A good analogy someone once told me was 'having a retained reflex is like a shopping trolley with a broken wheel. You really have to work at keeping the trolley straight'. Imagine the retained reflex is the broken wheel and your infant has to work so hard to stay on track (conform to 'normal' expectations), in addition to everything else they are learning to do – no wonder they may have trouble concentrating or have 'ants in their pants'.

Seek help early on from a cranial osteopath or chiropractor experienced in working with babies if the baby has experienced any trauma, a difficult birth or medical intervention, to check for any structural or neurological issues in the neck or spinal cord. If you have any concerns about development or if behaviour becomes an issue as your child grows, have their reflexes checked out (see page 189 for a chart summarising the emergence and integration of reflexes). It is a safe and less invasive starting point than other possible solutions. Have your baby or infant assessed by a trained therapist specialising in reflexes. Check the resources page 187 for where to seek help.

EARLY MOVEMENT

The womb provided a great training ground for movement to develop and connections to be made.

In utero kicks are a form of resistance training; mechanical stimulation which enhances bone density and growth.[13] We know that babies are born with immature bones, muscles, nervous system and more, so it is vitally important that they are moved and given every opportunity to move after birth. So let the kicks continue.

As your baby spends time on the floor, on both their back and front, they can explore their body more. Each kick on the floor tells them where their leg ends, how long they are, how much effort and movement is required to touch and push the floor, and the feel of textures beneath. Even in their crib or cot, they need their feet free to move.

Clothing should not restrict their movement either, even right down to their little toes. Those convenient stretch'n'grow jumpsuits, tights, and even socks can squash their toes without us knowing, and it's hard to grip with covered toes. I had a favourite little suit for one of my sons, and as he grew I unpicked the ends – so this is my suggestion to all parents now! That being said, one mum I know pointed out that when buying clothes for her daughter, she found most outfits on offer were dresses with tights. On warm days it was ok to just wear the dress but in winter she then had to buy boys' trousers to allow her daughter to be barefoot and warm!

It is really important to make sure your baby's socks and clothing are loose enough for their toes **in any position you have your baby**, including being carried in a sling. Take time to check next time you pick your baby up that their toes are still free. When I pick up babies wearing jumpsuits or tights in class or with friends I find myself having to adjust and pull down their clothes frequently to stop their wee toes from being totally crammed and squashed!

Back to movement, awareness of their inner self and where they are in space is important and all experimental movement helps develop their motor skills to be more coordinated. This is the start of 'pre-activation' whereby movement becomes familiar and muscle and tissue response is unconscious.

We can help our baby by doing gentle movements with them. Here's a few to get you started.

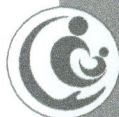

PASSIVE MOVEMENTS

Use this QR code to visit the resources page of my website, where you can view a video of the following movements. These are passive (you move them) movements you can do at any age with your baby. The range of movement will vary depending on age. You should NEVER force the movement. Tend to your baby's needs first as there is little point doing anything if they are hungry, tired or unsettled.

The benefits of these movements go beyond just the physical. You will be educating them about parts of their body by using the names of the body parts you are moving

and those you are moving towards. Find your own words or sounds to describe the movements and use rhymes or songs to make it more fun and memorable. We'll start with the legs and feet, of course, with baby lying on their back.

CARE: IF YOUR BABY HAS BEEN DIAGNOSED WITH HIP INSTABILITY OR DYSPLASIA CONSULT WITH YOUR PAEDIATRICIAN BEFORE DOING ANY OF THESE LEG MOVEMENTS.

Feet

- **ROLLING TOES:** hold their big toe between your thumb and first finger. Gently move it up and down and then roll it left and right. This is a very small movement. Do this with each toe.
- **PUSHING FEET:** put your palms on the soles of both feet and play a pushing game. Follow the movement of their legs or guide them up and down, around in circles (avoid if there is a hip problem) or just hold still and see if you can feel their toes moving on your palm as they explore.
- **ANKLE CIRCLES:** hold above your baby's ankle with one hand and with the other gently point their toes, then take their toes towards their knees. Explore what other movement they will let you do, such as circles, soles turning inwards.

Legs

- **KNEES UP:** holding your baby's legs above the ankle, gently push their knees into their tummy then relax back down. You can add a clockwise circular movement or a side-to-side sway when the knees are up.

- **CYCLING**: alternate pushing each knee into their tummy.
- **RELAX**: cradle one leg between both of your hands and bounce the leg up and down. See if they will let go so their leg goes heavy. Use words such as 'relax' and 'let go'. Praise them when they let go.

Arms
- **HUG**: hold baby's hands and bring their arms across their chest, alternating which arm is closest to the head each time. As they get older, their hand will reach over to the opposite shoulder. You can also do one arm at a time.
- **STARS**: again holding baby's hands, have them reach above their head (reach for the stars!), both arms together and then alternate one at a time. Make a star by taking the arms out to the sides at different angles to their body. Each time bring their arms back to their sides, tummy or chest.
- **NOSE TOUCH**: alternate movements of their arms and hands towards their nose or mouth.

Integrating
- Hold the left ankle and the right hand/wrist and bring them together over baby's tummy. This can be with either straight arms/legs or bend the knee so the hand touches the knee. Repeat on the other side.
- Guide one hand towards their opposite cheek, repeat with the other arm.
- Holding their ankles, cross their legs over each other and back, repeat with the other leg on top.
- Place your palms on your baby's sole and gently pulse back and forth so that their head nods up and down as you pulse.

The cross-crawl action is great for helping lay the foundations for the alternating movement required in crawling and walking. Actions that cross the midline of the body help integrate the left and right hemi-spheres of the brain.

Take the opportunity at bath time and when changing their nappy to play with these movements. At other times observe their movements knowing that what they are doing is training for the next stage of development. Inside the connections are being laid down. We can help unleash their potential.

Helping your child develop their central nervous system through movement, opportunity and interacting with them lays the foundations for the milestones ahead.

CHAPTER 4

EARLY MILESTONES: HEAD CONTROL, TUMMY TIME AND ROLLING

A WORD ON MILESTONES

Physical milestones are significant events for all parents. Milestones are visible, easily measured and can show how your infant is growing and developing, and as a parent we want to know our baby is on track.

However, there is a lot of variation and often wide timeframes regarding what happens when. For example, many books and websites will say 'around four to six weeks ...' or 'by about nine months ...'. The reason for this is because each infant's experience is different, and the opportunities and stimulation they receive are all different. Culture, environment, clothing and interactions with others all influence stages of development.

In the first two years, we see accelerated growth and development compared to other stages in life. Growth is individual and unique. Development is the result of interaction between maturation and learning.

And remember, earlier development or reaching milestones is not necessarily better.

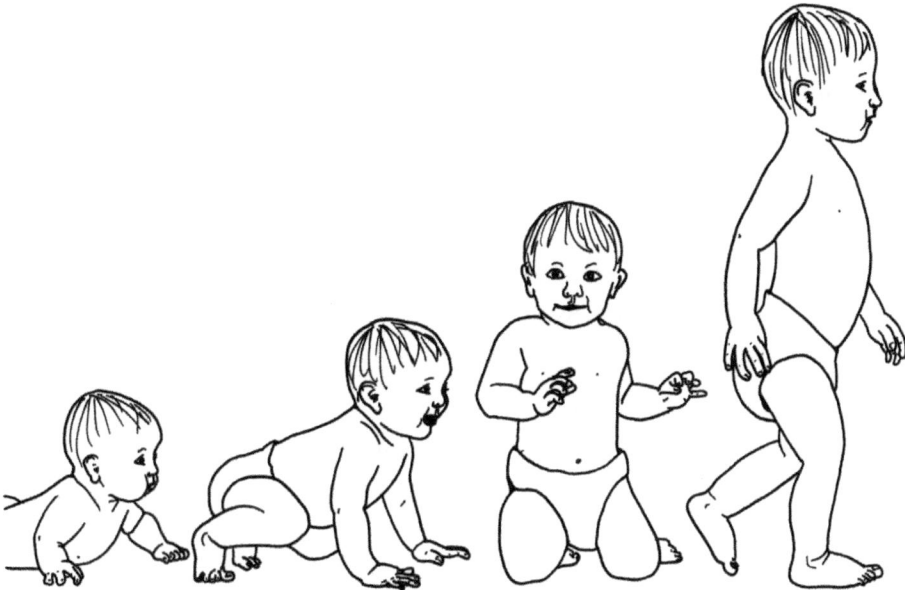

Head control is the beginning of your baby's independent movement. Only after achieving this can your baby then progress through the remaining physical milestones.

The patterns of growth and development are continuous, with a definite pattern: head to hips, toes to trunk, and from the centre outwards. A baby is born first equipped with reflexes, then gross motor skills come before fine motor skills and language – simple before more complex, which makes sense.

This progression gradually reduces the baby's base of support and at the same time increases their ability to move. They move from horizontal whole body on the ground to eventually up on two feet, from lifting their head to walking.

Movement and sensory input are definitely food for the brain, so you have the opportunity to both influence your baby's 'food' and even change your family's diet. Our world has become easier and easier, more comfortable, flatter and controlled – not a great diet. You don't need any special equipment to achieve this change; in fact, the fewer 'gadgets' you use, the better your baby's opportunity to develop in the way they are naturally meant to. In this book, I've broken down the milestones by the sequence they are attained rather than age as every child is different. Each has a suggested timeframe that you can check against, which is a collation of data from many resources. Use this as a guide only.

Each milestone is valuable so do not rush them. As they achieve each stage, your baby will be laying down the all-important neural connections, their central nervous system will be maturing, and their primitive reflexes will be integrating. If you try to move your baby on too soon, you may bring about a sense of frustration, even failure, for them. They may also adopt inappropriate strategies and miss vital learning.

The sweet success of walking comes from practice and mastering different skills along the way. Crawling provides your infant the opportunity to move and explore at ground level, and reach objects and people. Once walking, the whole room comes into view. Their world opens up more, and they can carry things.

We do not need to teach them how to move. Their body is wired to move with systems to create movement and stop movement. Primitive and postural reflexes are their 'tools of the trade' as Sally Goddard-Blythe wrote in her book *The Well Balanced Child*. We just need to provide every opportunity and a safe environment, and being footloose and footwear-free will help.

HEAD CONTROL

The first physical milestone that you might read about is head control. Until your baby has head control, it is important that during any movements, such as being lifted or put down, your baby's head is supported. It takes up to three months for them to be able to show some signs of control; full control appears at around five months of age.

At birth, the skull makes up about 25% of a baby's overall length and weight. To put that weight in perspective for you, I weigh around 60 kg and the average adult head weighs 5 kg. But if I were to imagine I had the same proportions as a newborn, my head would weigh more like 15 kg. If I lay down with a 10 kg bag of flour on my head and tried to get up, I think I would struggle! Give me a few months of training to develop more strength in my neck and maybe I could.

Like all other joints in their bodies, your baby has spaces (fontanelles) between individual bones in their skull which gives them greater flexibility to squeeze through the birth canal. The five skull bones fuse over time and the spaces close.

After birth, your baby's skull and body can be influenced by the positions they adopt, the surfaces they are placed upon, or the length of time they are in one position. For example, positional plagiocephaly (a flattening of one area of a baby's head) may result if your baby's head always rests a certain way. The result being the back or side of their skull, including facial bones, adapt through pressure and become flat and deformed.

The guidelines for safe sleep and prevention of SIDS (sudden infant death syndrome) recommend placing a baby on their back for sleep.[14] But if the baby is also placed in similar daytime positions (e.g., floor, change table, car seat, swing, pushchair), they will lack the variety of positioning to ensure they grow and develop optimally. We must give the brain every opportunity to grow inside without pressure from the outside, so it is crucial that parents following the 'back is best' sleeping guidelines ensure their baby is moved into different positions throughout the day.

Head control precedes balance and all other movements, and as your baby is mastering their head, other gross motor skills are emerging. The Landau and tonic labyrinthine reflexes both contribute to gaining control.

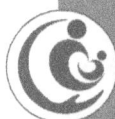

HELPING YOUR BABY GAIN HEAD CONTROL

- Use different objects, toys and noises to attract their attention, encouraging them to turn their head.
- Change the way you place them on the play mat so they can see different things: light from windows, shadows.
- If bottle-feeding, change the side you hold them during each feed.
- Carry them more, using a sling rather than using prams, buggies and car seats.
- Massage their scalp, neck and back.
- And of course, time on the floor on BOTH their back and tummy.

TUMMY TIME

Tummy time is vital for your baby's healthy development for a variety of reasons. The World Health Organisation recommend just thirty minutes spread throughout a day for better health and development outcomes.[15] You have no doubt been told tummy time is important. Studies confirm this and list a range of benefits, from earlier and improved head control to reducing the chance of obesity. [16]

Newborns have spent nine months in the womb, the last few being curled up in a ball, known as the 'fetal position'. When placed facedown, newborns may still adopt this flexed posture, bringing their knees up under their pelvis. This is the symmetrical tonic neck reflex (see page 39).

Lying facedown on the floor, the asymmetrical tonic neck reflex (see page 37) should kick in and help your baby turn their head so they can breathe. Your baby improves their head control by practicing lifting and turning it, driven by sights and sounds. You could say that your baby's vision and hearing drives them to move and explore.

It's not easy to go from the fetal position to flat on the floor, so take time with your baby to introduce tummy time.

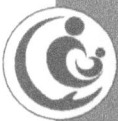

SOME POSITIONS TO INTRODUCE EARLY TUMMY TIME

- Lay your baby over your lap so their arms and legs are free.
- Lay your baby on your chest while you recline, lying on your back.
- Hold your baby tummy down on your arm while carrying them, resting their head by your elbow, your hand firmly holding between their legs, and their arms hanging either side of yours.

After one month or so, they should be able to lift their head for a moment. With practice lying on their tummy for short spells, by three months of age, they should have more control and be able to lift and hold their head. This gradual introduction to tummy time will build the tolerance and acceptance needed for baby to grow accustomed to tummy time. Rush it or leave them there too long and they will tell you. Short, frequent spells on their tummy is best. Why not join them? Grunts, groans and grizzles are to be expected as they lift and move this large part of themselves.

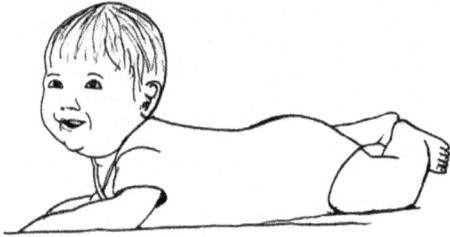

IMAGE 4.1: Time on their tummy helps develop neck extension.

Lying on their tummy helps develop their neck and back muscles. There is a band of extensor muscles either side of the spine running from the sacrum (a triangle-shaped bone at the base of the spine) up and connecting fascially over the top of the skull. When these muscles shorten they help lift up your baby's heavy head (IMAGE 4.1).

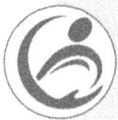

If you're not pregnant, head to the floor. Lying on your tummy try lifting your head, then your shoulders — without using your arms.

These back extensor muscles help unfold your baby from the flexed position in the womb and the position we cradle them in. The baby needs to balance and strengthen their front too, so they need to be moved regularly from their back to their front, and back again. Time on their back is also important for developing strength and control of their head. The floor is a safe place for your baby to practice what they need to.

So why else is tummy time important?

When your baby lifts and holds their head whilst on their tummy, this movement creates neck extension. This is a spinal curve that your baby needs for developing a healthy upright posture, for sitting and for walking.

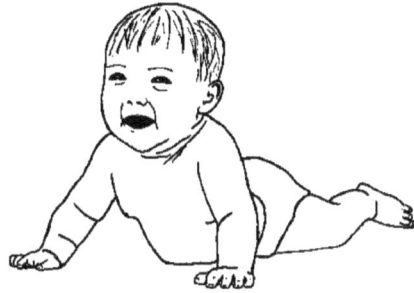

IMAGE 4.2: Pushing up with their arms develops their lumbar curve.

Tummy time also helps with developing arm strength and shoulder mobility. Your baby will practice pushing up to see what is happening in the world around them, reach out for toys, pull themselves forward (commando crawl) and even push themselves backwards. Pushing up with their arms helps develop their lumbar curve in the lower spine, which is another essential spinal curve (IMAGE 4.2).

Whilst your baby may complain and grizzle about being placed on their tummy, it is about building pathways and thresholds (think back to the hot tarmac/sand example, page 26). Before long, they will only want to be on their front. It is from this position that they can access moving, crawling, climbing and standing before they have the ability to walk. And it's a great position for future temper tantrums!

Tummy time helps integrate many of the primitive reflexes and accelerate the onset of belly crawling, pivoting and finally crawling.

On their front, your baby will have more opportunity, and perhaps more drive through their eyes, for movement and changing the relationship between their head, pelvis and ribs. These are all key aspects of walking and for when the symmetrical tonic neck reflex reappears so that they have the strength to push up onto their knees and rock back and forth.

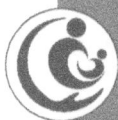

TOP TIPS FOR TUMMY TIME

As newborns

- Free feet (from clothing/footwear) and hands for exploring.
- Vary the environment: carpet, hard floor or grass.
- Place toys and objects at different distances for looking at and reaching for.
- Use a mirror or tactile play mat.
- Pick a spot by a window that creates shadows that move on the floor.
- Put a rolled towel or pillow under their chest with their arms free.
- Get down on the floor with them and play, chat and sing.
- Stroke their back using your full hand from top of head to their bottom like you would a cat; fingers down either side of the spine from neck to bottom.

As they get older

- Encourage reading or looking at pictures whilst lying on their tummy.
- Play games like blowing ping-pong balls across the floor.

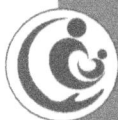

BASICS FOR BACK TIME ON THE FLOOR

As newborns

- Again, have the feet free.
- Hanging mobiles provide both visual and tactile stimulation with objects hanging within reach.

- Once they have found their feet, place loose socks on and let them pull them off.
- This a great time to start a massage! See the activity box on page 182 for tips on leg massage.

As they get older
- Get outdoors and lie down under trees, or on grass slopes watching clouds.
- Combine both positions and incorporate their vestibular system by finding gentle slopes to roll down.

Remember to gradually build their tolerance and always supervise them. Better still, join them and play.

A principal of two early childcare centres in the West Midlands, United Kingdom, shared a story with me about a young mother who brought her two-year-old daughter to the centre to be enrolled. The infant had been kept in a pushchair for most of her short life causing many developmental problems. 'I shall never forget the horror of leg braces and how the skills of walking, that we take for granted, had to be learnt, one minute part at a time.' The centre staff worked hard with the infant, in a programme of intensive activities both indoors and out. They 'transformed her life and life chances'. Sadly, the curvature in her spine remained, all easily preventable if only the child had been encouraged to move more in those important early few months.

Lying on their tummy, your baby may follow a sound, or you as you move, or reach up with an arm and look up at their hand in the air. With the weight of their head they may flip over onto their back! Or they may drive this movement from their legs or pelvis and, voila, they are rolling! And if, when you have been moving them from lying on their back to front and back again, you have rolled them, this movement will be familiar to them.

ROLLING

Chances are the first time your baby rolls it's a surprise, perhaps as a result of them arching their back and stiffening their body as seen with the backward TLR response (page 42). And whilst most will roll from tummy to back first, be ready for the unexpected! Your baby likely hasn't thought about how to roll; they just followed an object or sound, turned their head, an arm pushed up, their spine twisted and then woohoo – over they went. They will need help to get back to their tummy so they can practice, and watch their cues as after a couple of times they may have had enough (IMAGE 4.3).

To roll from their back to tummy may happen in two stages. During the first, they may roll onto their side as they practice flexing their legs and curl into almost a ball, similar to the fetal position in the womb. This may happen as they find their feet with their hands! And once on their side, they need to work out that they have to then extend by using their back muscles and straighten their legs to fully roll over, and bring their arms up in front. Or

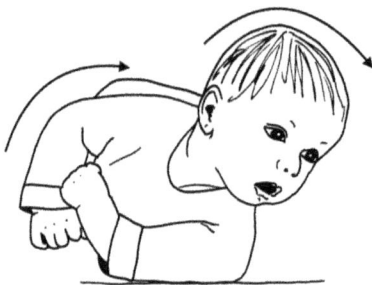

IMAGE 4.3: Over they go, rolling from tummy to back.

at the head end, their eyes or ears will be driving the movement. Their head may turn to look and, having developed great neck extension, they can keep looking until the rest of their body just has to follow **(IMAGE 4.4)**.

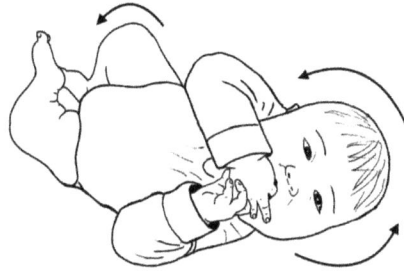

IMAGE 4.4: Neck extension helps with rolling from back to tummy.

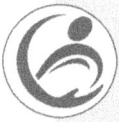

I encourage you to get on the floor and try rolling back and forth. Try different ways. Use your upper body to drive the movement allowing the lower body to follow effortlessly, then try using your legs to drive the movement. Explore what you need to be able to do to get your arms out of the way to stop yourself face-planting.

The key to rolling is giving them something to roll towards, bribery if you like! And don't be upset if your baby forgets how to do it for a few days. Understand that your baby may need to practice certain components to make good brain–body connections before they've completely got their rolling badge!

Rolling is a great manoeuvre for stimulating the vestibular system, helping develop balance and muscle tone through movement.

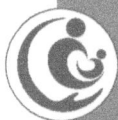

MOVEMENTS TO INTRODUCE ROLLING

- When picking your baby up off their back, roll them over a little, almost spiralling them (this also takes some strain off their neck).
- Gently push both knees into their tummy and roll baby onto their side; do both ways.
- Help them roll from their back to front and vice versa.
- Get down and roll around the floor (ignoring the dust under the sofa)!

As the signs of rolling appear, ensure your baby is safe, especially when on a bed or change table. In fact, once your baby starts rolling, it may be easier to change your baby's nappy on the floor, and this becomes part of your own movement regime to move more.

Floor time with space to move and explore is crucial for letting these skills develop. Limit time spent in 'man-made' devices that restrict free movement to when you really need them. When your baby is on the floor, make sure their feet are naked and free so they can help. If they grizzle and cry, check it's not because they are frustrated or stuck; in other words, don't be in a rush to pick them up. Help them over – if they still cry then pick them up. Lastly, get down with them – it'll do you the world of good!

CHAPTER 5

SITTING AND CRAWLING

REMEMBER MATURITY AND PHYSICAL MILESTONES DO NOT always relate to age.

Your baby's physical growth contributes to reaching milestones. From newborn to two years of age, your baby's length doubles with the rest of their body bringing balance to their oversized head. At birth, their centre of mass is at the bottom of their breastbone and as they develop it shifts down to just above their belly button. Whilst development affects the shift, the location of their centre of mass affects their movement.

If you think about the 'growth curve' in your baby health book, it is not an accurate way of depicting what actually happens. Growth does not happen along a steady curve. It could be better described as 'growth spurts' whereby it accelerates at times and moves more slowly at others.[17] The rate of growth may also influence how your baby's movement develops, as they have to adjust to the new length, width or weight. Increased hunger, unsettled behaviour and altered sleep patterns can all be attributed to growth spurts.

Development of movements are, as I have mentioned, an individual process and also happens in spurts. Your baby has so much going on as their vision improves and sounds and words start forming, no wonder they have to sleep so much. Your baby needs time and repetition to learn and discover efficiencies. Movement is goal-based, they do have a plan, and most importantly they enjoy it.

Your baby will reach the milestones and develop in the timeframe right for them, provided they are given opportunity to. If you have concerns at any stage, consult your healthcare professional.

SITTING

As we progress through the stages of development, sitting is a position in which we often first observe an upright posture.

Infants can be propped up in a sitting position once they have good head control but doing this serves little purpose in helping them to learn how to get there.

It is important to limit time sitting in man-made supports such as pushchairs, swings, bouncers, moulded seats and car seats. These devices will not help strengthen the muscles needed for sitting and they generally keep baby's lower spine in a flexed position (think about the earlier story of the child kept in a pushchair). Pulling their hands to bring them into a sitting position does little to help them learn also.

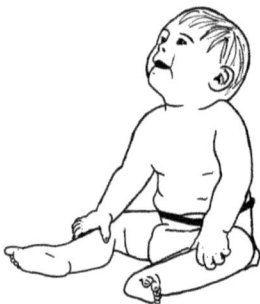

IMAGE 5.1: The floor provides a safe place to practice sitting and falling.

The floor offers space for free movement of their hips and legs, encouraging their own inbuilt natural support (IMAGE 5.1). Sitting is your baby's first vertical experience in gravity (apart from being held when carried or sitting on your lap) and it stimulates the vestibular system in preparation for moving into a more upright world.

Every milestone has progressions. Your baby must learn to get to a sitting position by themselves. You can encourage them but try not to assist them too much. Remember they are laying neural pathways and building strength.

Rolling brings a spiralling action into the body, which can lead to sitting. Sitting requires your baby to be able to roll both ways, use upper body strength, have the ability to shift their weight left and right, forwards and backwards whilst maintaining good head control.

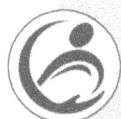

Try for yourself, move from your tummy (if not pregnant) and then your back exploring what body parts you need to move and support. How many different ways can you move from the floor into a seated position?

Moving from being horizontal to vertical requires a whole-body effort.

Your baby needs the variety in movement that learning to sit brings not just for developing the strength and stability for the next milestones but for integrating those all-important primitive reflexes.

As they sit, they can explore their feet, their genitals (having had boys I can vouch for this one!) and how far they can reach. They may topple over, so make sure their space is clear of sharp and hard objects. This is an opportunity for your baby to start experience falling. Yes, falling! Falling is part of your baby's vestibular and response training.

Ideally, your baby would be sitting on the floor throughout their infancy as once they enter the world of institutions, they will spend enough time sitting on chairs! Floors provide variety and freedom

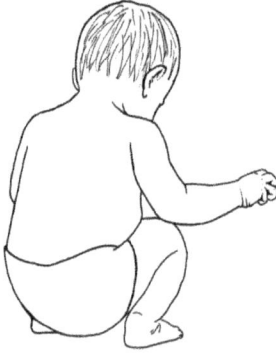

IMAGE 5.2: Squatting is a great position for sitting and transitioning to walking.

to sit or squat in more natural ways to keep their joints flexible and body strong.

It would appear that as adults our movement diminishes over time through lack of having to move a certain way, our lifestyles and our culture. As children, we spend years learning to move, play, and use the full range of our bodies, and then as adults we lose these opportunities as different priorities and expectations of adulthood become important – but at what cost?

Katy Bowman, author and biomechanist, wrote 'we have shaped an entire science to make sense of our culture's lack of particular movements'.[18] To give you an example, your baby is born with at least 60 degrees of ankle (dorsi) flexion[19] – the action your ankle joint makes when you do a squat (IMAGE 5.2). This gradually reduces to between 35 and 40 degrees as the bones, joints and soft tissues mature, but the normal range of ankle movement in adults when standing has been established as 7 to 35 degrees – that is a huge range.[20] By saying this is 'normal', is society accepting that it's ok to have less? After all, we only need 10 degrees of movement for walking.

Sitting on the floor will encourage your baby to keep moving their feet and joints, and help their body to be adaptable as they adopt different positions. Sitting also opens up more opportunities for play and stimulation. So once they can sit don't go rushing out to buy those cute table and chairs, invest in a jungle gym!

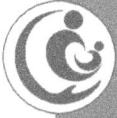

I do wonder if infants who spend more time propped up to sit and placed in sitting devices have more of a tendency to adopt the bum-shuffle and scoot movement as a way of getting around rather than coming up from the floor to crawl.

Learning to sit for themselves is a great launchpad for crawling.

CRAWLING

There are mixed thoughts about crawling and whether it's an essential milestone. I am hoping that you may now see that crawling is needed and a necessary movement for reflex integration and brain development, and that given every opportunity to progress through the sequential learning patterns that are innate it will happen.

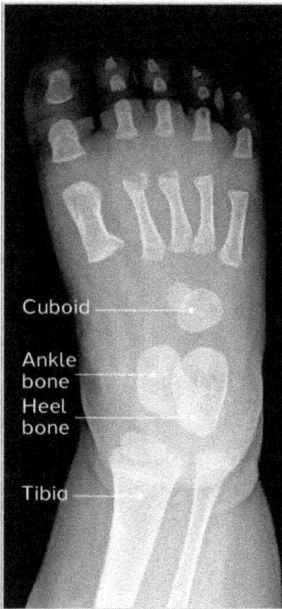

IMAGE 5.3: X-ray view looking from the sole upwards of a six-month-old baby's right foot.

Labels on image: Cuboid, Ankle bone, Heel bone, Tibia

Spending time on their tummy combined with the symmetrical tonic neck reflex brings your baby onto their hands and knees. Then time spent rocking helps them gain control so that they can move the rest of their body independently from their head. This is key for advancing to crawling forwards. So, head down-bum up is your baby working hard!

Crawling requires coordinated movement of their limbs and more movement through their joints, so let's pause a moment to look at joints.

JOINTS

Joints give us the ability to move. Where bones meet, you get a joint. A joint is commonly defined as 'two parts of the skeleton fitted together' or 'a place in the body where two bones are connected, attached',[21] all somewhat implying that bones touch.

Check out the X-ray of a six-month-old infant's foot (IMAGE 5.3). We can see vast spaces between the dots of immature foot bones, but because we know fascia is everywhere, we know these spaces are created by our fascial system, designed to keep the bones apart allowing for future bone growth and, more importantly, movement.

Another view of joints is that they are 'the areas where two or more bones meet. Most joints are mobile, allowing the bones to move.'[22] I like this one better. Joints are there to guide and define movement.

None of your infant's bones are fully formed at birth and are not fully developed until their late teens. This means neither are their joints, which is why movement, particularly varied movement, is crucial throughout their young life and beyond. To keep their joints healthy, they need to explore their own unique movements daily. So let's get moving ... **(IMAGE 5.4)**

The first independent movement of crawling (though you could argue that rolling is their first) helps build strength, spatial awareness and confidence. Exploring their surrounds opens up your baby's world (whilst providing new challenges for parents). Crawling requires the left and right sides of the body to work together, which provides a more active integration of the left and right sides of the brain, beyond the passive movement you did with them as a baby.

IMAGE 5.4: Crawling creates a side bending movement with ribs and hips doing opposite movements.

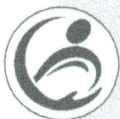

Your baby will progress from four, to three and finally their first experience of life on two supports as the opposite hand and knee/foot are on the ground whilst the other hand and knee/foot travel forward through the air. Your baby's upper and lower body also do opposite movements creating a side bend at their waist. The movement looks very similar to the spinal Galant reflect (page 40), doesn't it?

Balance is also challenged, and soon they realise they are stable with three points of contact when they pause to reach for objects. Shoulder stability and strength improves, combined with the reaching for objects, all helping the development of fine motor skills.

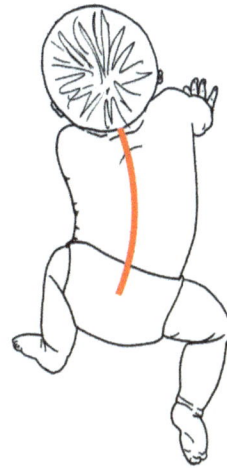

The best way to understand crawling is to get down and try it. Start in a lying position on the floor, then from sitting. Hopefully your body remembers what to do, or do you have to think about which arm and leg to lift first?

Some infants may bum-shuffle, scoot, bum-jump or completely skip crawling all together. Whilst these variations in mobility may seem to be the answer for some, often they are one-sided movements. For example an infant will often scoot one way, using the same leg and arm all the time, the spine only moving/flexing to one side. These asymmetrical movement patterns may lead to unbalanced structural development such as scoliosis, and poor coordination in the years to come. Also look out for the subtle knee/foot crawl when they use one knee and the other foot. The asymmetrical adaptions may also impair the integration of the symmetrical tonic neck reflex, potentially leading to other developmental delays or issues.

I believe that crawling should be encouraged due to the cross-crawl contralateral action of the limbs which is then taken into walking. The practice of coordinated movement with the safety net of being lower to the ground and on all fours helps develop muscle tone and balance, which stimulates the vestibular system and improves hand-eye coordination. Up in the brain, connections are stronger between the two hemispheres.

Crawling is also a whole-body movement from the superficial layers of the skin, through the fascia and right down to the bones and organs. Everything moves because everything is connected.

Down at the feet, bear crawling especially requires toe extension (bending them back) for extra grip and push forwards (IMAGE 5.5). Your baby may crawl with their toes flat but they will soon realise the usefulness of the toes when they move from all fours to upright. The plantar reflex is still present during the crawling stage and should disappear with the use of the toes. Bare feet are best to allow for the toes to work.

This first form of independent movement requires route planning and potential problem-solving as your baby manoeuvres themselves to get where they want, hence

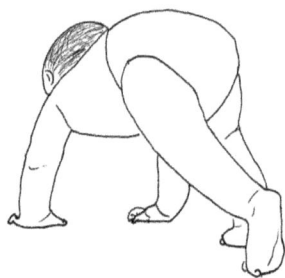

IMAGE 5.5: Bear crawling uses their toes more.

both sides of their brain having to work together. With every successful journey, your baby's confidence will grow.

Discovering and reaching places by crawling under and over objects, forwards and backwards and, like a bear, on hands and feet will all serve them both physically and mentally. Why not join them?

Remember it's not just about being able to crawl and then moving on to the next milestone, time spent crawling is so important for both cognitive and behavioural development.

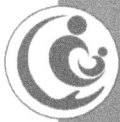

STRATEGIES TO HELP ENCOURAGE A MORE COORDINATED WAY OF MOVING

- Get down and crawl with them; they may copy your movement.
- Try supervised stair climbing to encourage coming forward onto hands and knees.
- Create small obstacle courses with pillows or small heights that they have to climb over, or a course with chairs and low tables they have to go under – again encouraging use of the crawling action.
- Place staggered mats that they have to place their hands and knees/feet on.
- Praise them when they move using both sides of their body.
- Have crawling races as they get older.
- Try different styles of crawling: commando or bear.

CHAPTER 6

STANDING, SQUATTING AND CLIMBING

CRAWLING OPENS UP A WHOLE NEW WORLD TO YOUR INFANT. Now they have the ability to reach places they once only dreamt of going, seeing around the corner, following you and others, chasing the cat or dog – oh, the joys!

And then they learn that with this new freedom they can balance on knees and one hand whilst reaching up to the top of the coffee table, and next thing you know they are standing and the TV remote is fair game.

It's important to keep in mind that this new skill is a long way from walking; after all it's their very first solo venture into being upright in gravity.

PULL UP AND STAND

I remember going in to Nick's room hearing he was awake and there he was, standing in his cot squealing with delight and bouncing up and down using his knees. Pulling to stand offers a natural transition from one position to another, and requires involvement of your infant's entire body and mind. Your infant will reach up, and then adopt a semi-kneeling position as they find their balance and push through one foot to lift their body and free the other leg to follow suit. Down at the foot, the ankle must bend, feet push into the ground, toes grip and receptors send messages to the brain.

Or your infant may go from the bear crawl position, squat, reach up for support and come up to standing. Your infant will be discovering the effort required to move with the gravitational force pushing down on them and making use of ground force reaction by pushing their feet downwards **(IMAGE 6.1)**.

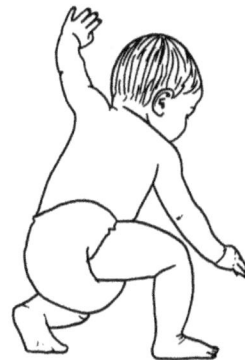

IMAGE 6.1: Using the support of the wall your baby pushes through both feet, all joints are involved and up they go.

Celebrate this supported standing and allow time in this stage to move from the various floor positions to vertical. Allow your baby time to work out the various ways they can come to standing, with and without support or help.

This is the first time your infant's feet support their entire weight and they will be testing the relationships between their heavy head, centre of mass, gravity and feet. Sensory and proprioceptive information from their feet is crucial so being barefoot is optimum.

This loading of the feet will kick off their body laying down the layers of dense fascia that will eventually be known as plantar fascia as the foot supports the weight of their body.

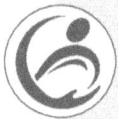

You guessed it – get down on the floor and crawl over to the kitchen table or bench. Reach up with one hand and then work out the various ways you can rise to stand. Now imagine you can't walk yet – what do you do next?

Stuck in standing, though delighted with themselves, what do they do next? A nappy makes for a soft landing – *plop*! – your infant has arrived at the next challenge of a controlled descent. Options may include a squat or reversing down on one knee, all requiring stability and full ranges of movement of all joints, a whole body event.

Once your baby has reached this stage ensure that their clothing does not get in the way by keeping the feet bare, as it will enable them to grip more and gain more confidence. They may also discover kneeling during this time.

SQUATTING

Squatting is a great transitional position and no doubt when your infant does it many times a day, you'll be wishing you could move with such easy flexibility. Encourage this position by not offering custom-built toddler chairs, which will ensure your infant retains great mobility of all joints (as discussed in the previous chapter) and develops the strength they need.

Squat to unassisted standing helps build strength and balance, and will become frequently used during walking.

Of course you need to think about safety around the home more now. It's time to shift objects to higher places or the remote to the middle of the coffee table. Be prepared for sticky fingers on the TV, fridge door and more!

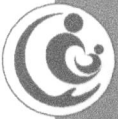

STRATEGIES TO HELP YOUR INFANT SQUAT AND STAND

- Place their favourite toys in different places where you don't mind them standing, like the coffee table.
- If they have bottles or drinking cups, place them where your child can stand, hold the table and grab a quick drink!
- Encourage your child to use their legs to stand before you pick them up.
- Hold off on buying infant chairs and cushions for them to sit on.
- Massage their legs and feet, back and arms.
- Get down and squat with them. Hold their hands and squat together.

CLIMBING

I often hear parents saying their infant climbed before they could walk, as if it is some extraordinary feat requiring advanced skills, thus questioning if it is normal or not. It is perfectly normal for an infant to climb before they can walk.

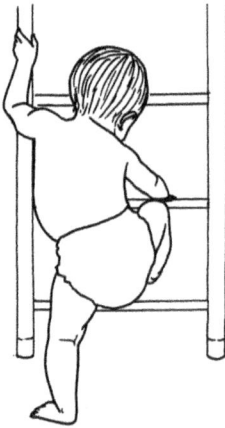

IMAGE 6.2: Climbing and crawling have similar movements of arms, legs and body.

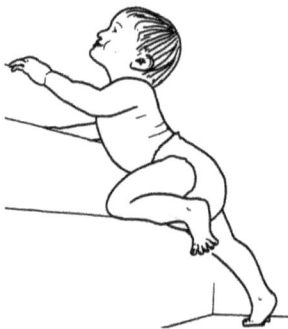

IMAGE 6.3: Climbing uses their toes and improves spatial awareness.

The combination of being able to crawl over to, say, a bookshelf and pull themselves to standing provides the perfect opportunity to crawl upwards! If your infant is more of a bum-shuffler or scooter, encouraging them to climb will help them gain some of the benefits that crawling brings.

Climbing requires the same contralateral and side-bending movement as crawling (IMAGE 6.2), and is a skill that helps further develop balance, hand-eye and limb coordination and overall strength. Your infant's hands will no doubt be bare, so free the feet; both are needed for grip. The toes definitely need to be free (IMAGE 6.3).

Climbing encourages more spatial awareness. Your infant needs to consider how far they have to lift their foot which they can't actually see, which in turn strengthens the neural pathways and proprioception. Climbing introduces a greater level of problem-solving and risk-taking which supports cognitive development and builds confidence.

And remember going up is one thing, how they come down is another. Don't be too quick to grab them (unless they are in danger of falling). Congratulate your infant for their climb and then guide them back down. You may find if you go to hold them they will completely let go and give you their weight; after all, they trust you. Guide their foot to the shelf/step/branch below, encourage them, allow them to take their time.

Inside your home, stairs, chairs, bookshelves, beds and cabinets are all appealing – trust me, I know! Ben, my second son, would often climb his high chair. I'd find him precariously poised, feet on the foot rest and holding on to the tray for dear life. Your backyard and local park also provide plenty of opportunities. Allow your infant to crawl, climb, and explore.

Be ready!

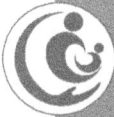

IDEAS FOR SAFE CLIMBING

- Safety proof your home with stair gates and secure climbable shelves to the wall.
- Create a 'climb-safe' zone for them to practice in. Pile pillows around the coffee table or at the bottom of a small shelf.
- Adopt different positions on the floor for them to climb over you. Grasping your clothes is quite different to a hard shelf or table and will prepare them for trees!
- Adapt their obstacle course from the crawling stage using higher objects such as chairs to climb over (keeping their safety in mind).
- Use a chair, step stool or specially designed standing tower for your infant to join you at the kitchen bench.
- Visit the local playground, allow them to crawl around (barefoot of course, if it's safe) and find things to pull themselves up on and even climb.

I do wonder if those that climb early do so because they are presented with opportunities earlier than others. I am always amazed at how infants appear to have no fear. Inbuilt instinct drives them. Their learning is limitless, however, as adults are we the ones who put the brakes on, conditioning them out of their free state and perhaps even instilling fear in them?

Time spent crawling, squatting, standing (supported) and climbing is loading their bones, making them stronger, developing muscles and tensional lines – the body's puppet strings. This is all preparation for walking, so don't rush them. Let's check out their developing body in preparation for walking.

POSTURE AND CURVES

Looking at the body from a side view (sagittal plane) shows the upright standing posture as one of curves. Your baby slowly unfolds from a curved fetal position at birth to being upright, from a C-shaped spine to an upright undulating one with curves. Through tummy time and early movement, as discussed already, your baby will develop the all-important curves in the neck and lower back (IMAGE 6.4).

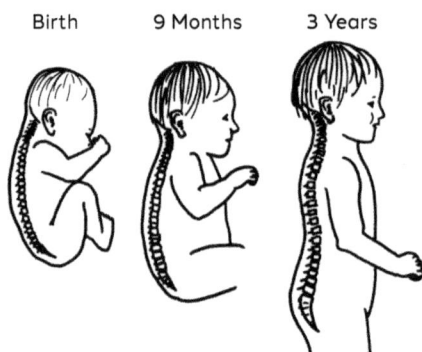

IMAGE 6.4: Stage of spinal development: from C-curve at birth to developing neck and lower back curves.

What is not shown in the image are the curves, or arches, that develop in the feet during this time. From skull to sole, your baby will evolve into a series of alternating curves, a deliberate design for strength and adaptability.

These spinal curves give greater flexibility and the ability to absorb shock. So do joints. For example, jumping requires the ankles, knees and hips all to bend on landing, absorbing some of the impact. The discs and curves of the spine also absorb the impact so that the brain is protected. Similarly, the curves (arches) in the feet are the first to absorb the impact with the bones opening on the underside and the foot lengthening and widening! Fascia is also a shock absorber.

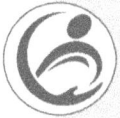

> Up you get – jump up and down a couple of times. When you stop, do you feel a ripple through your body? That's your fascia. Also notice that you don't jump with straight legs; the joints in your legs act to propel you and then absorb the impact.

Healthy upright posture, a position to move from, requires the undulating flow of the curves, balance between front and back, left and right, from the feet up to the head.

As you observe your infant coming to standing, they will be negotiating with gravity to find this optimal position, all being well. I believe that it is the introduction of external influences, objects and our environments that over time compromises this balance and central place. One common posture that used to be only seen in adults was that of forward head posture, where the head is forward of the ribs and pelvis. With greater use of technology, younger and younger people are being observed with this posture, which some have even called it 'text-neck' (IMAGE 6.5). It is disturbing to see infants in pushchairs and car seats

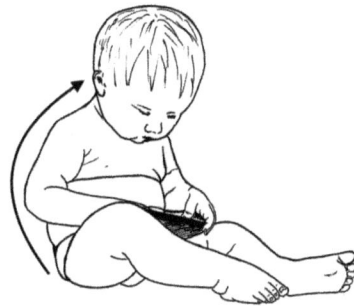

IMAGE 6.5: 'Text-neck': the entire spine is compromised and looks similar to the C-curve at birth, delaying the development of the neck and lower back curves.

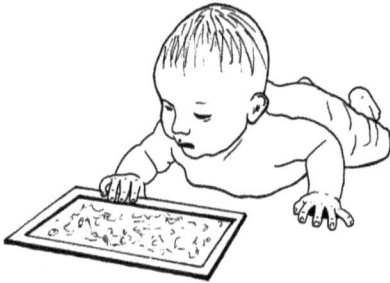

IMAGE 6.6: Lying on the floor to read or play goes some way to creating a healthy spine; changing positions frequently is also a great idea.

looking down at the device they are holding, instead of engaging with the people and the world around them. A much better option for your infant reading a book or using a device is lying on the floor (IMAGE 6.6).

Upright postural alignment should also be viewed in terms of the connections and relationships between body parts, not in terms of isolated bones, joints and muscles. When you look at a tree you see a tree, every part of the tree connected.

And central to these relationships is fascia – fascia that connects and separates everything in the body, and gives us our shape. Slowly the message of the role and importance of fascia is trickling out to medical and health practitioners, movement and manual therapists. I firmly believe parents should have this knowledge too as you want the best for your child. Researchers are discovering more and more each day about the significance and meaning of fascia and turning the tables on previous models of anatomy. Now is the right time to further your knowledge, after all it's all about you too!

Rather than looking at body parts individually as muscles, joints and ligaments, let's imagine the continuities. Myofascia (myo = muscle) 'rubber bands' rise from the feet to encompass the back, front, sides, and insides of the body, wrapping and weaving continuously from one end to the other, balancing and supporting your infant as they push to stand. After all, there are no strings pulling your infant up. What I love about the body is its total interconnectivity and interactivity.

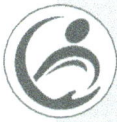

Stand up – now shift your pelvis to the right. Feel what happens in your feet as they have to adapt. There will be movement across the ankle joints, as the bones and soft tissues of the feet adjust their tone and tension to recalibrate. And your feet do this without you having to think about it – the wondrous integration of proprioception (where we are/how we move) and tension adjustment through the myofascial system, not to forget all the neural pathways. Scan the rest of your body – it all had to react to your pelvis moving.

Moving by way of adjusting tension in our body brings us nicely to the model of biotensegrity.

BIOTENSEGRITY

Let me introduce to you three gentlemen, Dr Stephen Levin, Kenneth Snelson and Buckminster Fuller: a surgeon, a sculptor and a systems theorist. They developed the conceptual framework of 'tensegrity' (tension + integrity).[23] Snelson was known for his sculptures (IMAGE 6.7); he used the description 'floating compression'. Fuller, with his mathematical background, coined the term 'tensegrity', and from there, in the 1980s, Dr Levin proposed 'biotensegrity' as a theory to understand biological

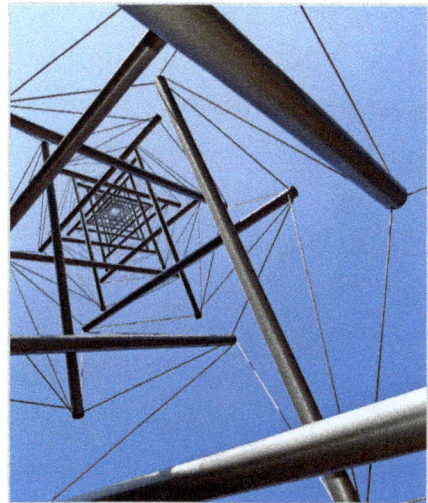

IMAGE 6.7: Kenneth Snelson's 'Needle Tower' (1968), a design of struts held apart by tension cables.

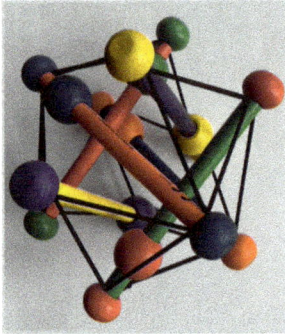

IMAGE 6.8: Manhattan Skwish Rattle, a child's version of Snelson's tower.

form, from the cellular level to whole organisms such as humans. Biotensegrity is a model of self-organisation.

The Manhattan Skwish Rattle child's toy (IMAGE 6.8) is an example of tensegrity in movement. It is made of elastic which provides the tension, compressing and holding the wood in place. Its three-dimensional form helps keep its structural integrity. At rest, tension and strain are distributed equally throughout the structure. If you push it down, it will bounce back. If you pull apart two struts, other struts will also move. If you pull or cut one piece of elastic, the whole structure will respond, both locally and globally.

In the body, bones are the compression elements and myofascia the tensional. With the small size of the foot muscles and the ropiness of tendons coming down into the foot, collectively they utilise tensioning (like pulling on the elastic) rather than strength to move.

The body has the ability to reshape and respond to strain by distributing it through the entire body. Movement in one part of the body affects other parts of the body – when your baby rolls, regardless of whether they initiated the movement at the head or legs, the twisting action brings the rest of the body with it. We can also observe this in primitive tonic neck reflexes (ATNR/STNR) with the position of the head initially driving the response of both arms and legs of your baby.

The human body is so cleverly designed: the packaging and wrapping, spaces and bones that allow for both support and freedom of movement from the feet and through the rest of the body.

When your infant learns to walk it's as if their foot is the puppeteer of their body; the movement of their bones tensions the cables (soft tissues) in both feet and lower legs to direct movement. All the neural connections from the eyes, ears and proprioceptors are vital for the puppeteer to perform, responding to their moving mass above and adapting in an instance.

It is important to see posture as a place or moment in time. As your infant practices standing, moving from one posture to another, one stable state to another, they will find their balance around a central position.

So as you observe your infant standing, swaying, supported in gravity, be mindful of what is required of them to get there. Not just bones and muscles, but also awareness of where they are in space and how they moved to get there (proprioception). Be mindful of the connection they need with the ground and remove all foreign barriers such as shoes.

CHAPTER 7

CRUISING AND THE NOVICE WALKER

IT IS HARD WHEN OTHER PARENTS SAY THEIR INFANT IS WALKING earlier than yours. Remember that your infant is unique and with the knowledge that you have now, you know that being hasty is not always a good thing. A solid, strong foundation and time taken to achieve all the milestones in their own time will serve them well going forward.

That being said, with this knowledge if you notice your child is not progressing then do not hesitate to seek professional advice. As with all the preceding milestones, your infant will need time, repetition and practice to master walking. Cruising is a great way to safely move in this vertical moving position.

CRUISING

The next step, or rather the first step, towards walking is from the standing position, holding on to something with both hands and taking a tentative step sideways.

Cruising around walls and furniture helps build strength and confidence. Whilst it is crab-like in motion, it is their first experience of lifting a foot and placing it a little further away from their centre, then shifting their weight to that foot so as to lift the other foot. All the time holding on to something solid, the hands are very much involved during this stage.

This sideways movement is potentially the start of laying down the iliotibial band (a band of thickened fascia on the side of the thigh) and strengthening the muscles on the side of the body. Remember we are more than just a back and front.

Cruising is also an important stage for helping improve balance and coordination, with a little extra problem-solving thrown in for good measure.

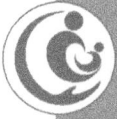

IDEAS TO SUPPORT CRUISING

- Resist the urge to grab their hand and help them walk.
- Provide clear pathways around furniture and walls; make a course for them to follow, changing the height of support to see if they can adapt.
- Place their favourite toys at one end of the sofa.
- Place pictures at their head height to look at as they move.
- As they become more confident, create gaps between furniture to challenge them to briefly move unsupported.
- Place small items on the floor for them to negotiate and step over.
- And of course, keep the feet naked for the best sensory input!

You may also find that your infant will drop down and crawl to get somewhere quicker. This mix'n'match of movement will continue until walking is established.

Your toddler is well on their way to walking in three dimensions, the three planes of motion that we move through. If you think back to your baby's tummy time and lying on their back, initially most actions of the legs and head were in the 'sagittal plane', e.g., when they pushed up their chest and head with their arms. Your baby then started rolling and turning their head; this rotating happens in the 'transverse plane'. Cruising, moving sideways, occurs in the 'frontal plane'. Your infant needs practice moving through all of these planes – bending, twisting, flexing and extending, in a variety of ways in preparation for walking.

THE NOVICE WALKER

It won't surprise you when I say 'infants don't walk like adults' and we now know each infant will develop at their own pace. The first phase of learning how to move upright in gravity lasts for three to six months, progressing from standing to cruising, to supported walking with the help of someone holding their hand, to finally independent walking. The second phase of fine-tuning happens over several years. Infants are often referred to during this time as 'toddlers', a word derived from 'to toddle', meaning to walk unsteadily (IMAGE 7.1).

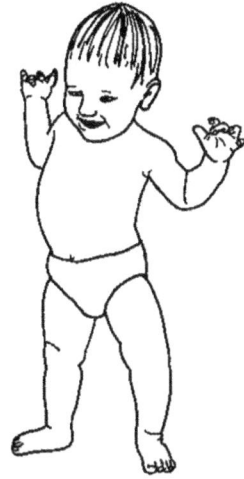

IMAGE 7.1: Unsteady first steps: the novice walker or toddler.

The characteristics of the onset of walking include:

- wider base of support, i.e., feet placed wide
- arms raised or outstretched
- slower, shorter steps with longer time spent in a split stance with both feet on ground
- lifting foot before placing, more knee flexion
- pausing every couple of steps.

These are learning strategies and assist with balance and coordination. You may be tempted to grab those wavering arms but hold back. Those arms are working hard at stabilising your toddler.

Toddlers rarely move in a straight line or continuously and they fall frequently, providing variability for their motor learning. It is therefore quite a challenge to assess a toddler walking, which limits research available on this topic. At New York University[24] researchers challenged the 'norm' when they found that it was potentially nappies causing the wider stance (IMAGE 7.2). All other research I reviewed never

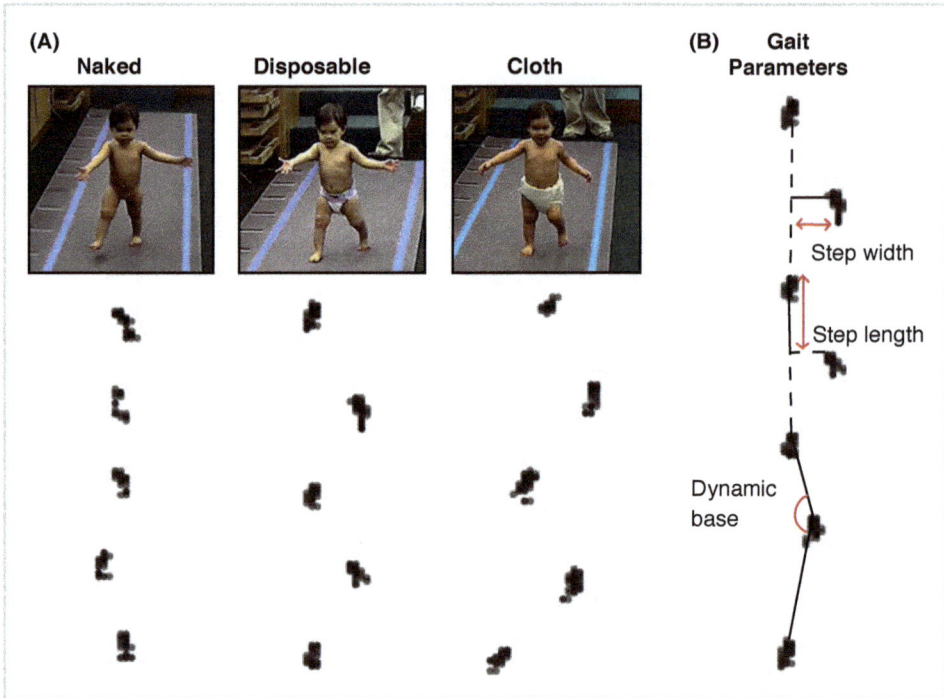

IMAGE 7.2: (A) Sample footprint paths from one typical infant walking while naked, wearing a disposable diaper, and wearing a cloth diaper. Infant is walking from top to bottom. Marks represent the pressure points of each footfall recorded by the gait carpet. (B) Gait parameters illustrated with footfalls recorded by the gait carpet as infant walked from top to bottom. Top: Step width is the side-to-side distance between feet. Middle: Step length is the front-to-back distance between consecutive footfalls. Bottom: Dynamic base is the angle between three consecutive steps. (Cole et al., 'Go Naked: Diapers Affect Infant Walking.' Image and caption republished with permission of John Wiley & Sons.).

reported on what toddlers were wearing. This suggests that perhaps the characteristic of the wide base of support is being influenced by an external device (nappy), so along with bare feet, a naked bottom may help with learning to walk. But I'll let you decide on that one!

When learning to walk, one function of the foot is to be adaptable, aiding with balance. The foot supports your toddler's bodyweight and absorbs impact, with the fat pad helping distribute load to protect the immature foot structure. The adapting, sensing foot acts as a messenger centre with its many receptors sending messages to their brain. Every sway, stumble, step and fall feeds information to their system. It is thought that the average toddler will take over 2,000 steps per hour with over fifteen falls a day on their way to becoming an expert walker.

In 'novice' walking, we don't see a heel strike, pronation (rolling inwards to flatten arch), to toe-off pattern as seen in adults. Instead there are a variety of ways your toddler may place their foot.[25]

FOREFOOT FIRST – forefoot, midfoot then heel (**IMAGE 7.3**).

FLAT FOOT – forefoot and heel placed simultaneously (**IMAGE 7.4**).

QUICK HEEL – quick contact with heel followed by rest of foot.

Regardless of your toddler's strategy, each will have a beneficial effect on the strengthening of their foot and supporting tissues. This is especially significant for the practice of the important action of toe-off (**IMAGE 7.5**) which is rehearsed with every step regardless of how the initial contact is made. As they come to the end of their stride (the moment when legs are furtherest apart), their back heel lifts, they roll through the foot and push forward through their big toe.

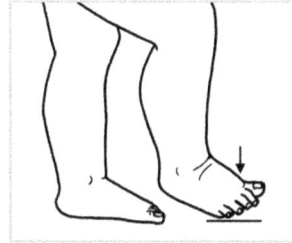

IMAGE 7.3: Forefoot landing.

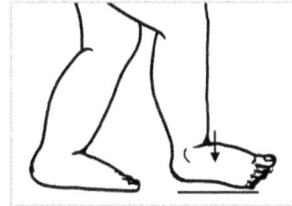

IMAGE 7.4: Flat foot landing.

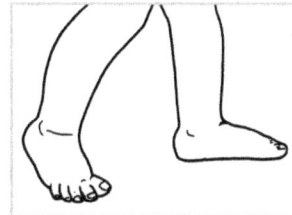

IMAGE 7.5: Toe-off, pushing off with the back leg to propel them forwards.

When I recall my son Nick starting to walk, the image I still have in my mind is that of someone onboard a ship in rough seas. He teetered left and then right, arms reaching out, feet going down to hit the deck but the deck was lower than he thought, so *bump*, he would end up falling. Then, as if not to be beaten by the ocean life, he would be up again. A drunk pirate also came to mind! Such a joyful moment for any parent or caregiver.

Walking has by some been described as 'controlled falling' and we may well be able to see this as toddlers totter, trying not to fall. Falling is an important part of learning, so managing the environment is important with removing or covering sharp table edges or providing a designated wide runway for practicing. Learning to fall safely and get up again is something that we, as adults, don't think about, let alone realise is part of training all those proprioceptors in the foot, ankle and up through their leg. Toddlers recover from the bumps and bruises much quicker than adults, after all they are much closer to the ground and therefore don't land as hard.

Once up on two legs your toddler will spend the next few years exploring life from this upright posture. All the wobbles and falls provide information about that place, where balance and alignment is achieved and optimal, a place they move from and back to.

As your toddler becomes more experienced, their balance increases, their arms relax and they discover they can carry things. Over time, their stance narrows (nappy dependent) and their stride length increases due to accessing more knee and hip extension. A heel strike should start to dominate their pattern.

At first, your toddler may appear bow-legged, as they become stronger they should straighten. They then may appear knock-knee'd – as if their legs have gone too far the other way from bowed – but this too over time should disappear.

Their flat-footed appearance will also resolve itself as loading stimulates bone growth to continue and muscles to adapt and strengthen. As their inside arch starts forming, pressure shifts from a midfoot focus to heel and forefoot – a tripod of support. Your toddler's foot becomes an adaptable shock pad and a catapult. This can take up to eight to ten years, so be patient. If you recall, with twenty-six bones in each foot creating thirty-three joints, that's a mountain of movement.

When learning to walk, your toddler's feet need stimulation from different surfaces and temperatures, and a variety of movement from uneven ground to inclines. The more your toddler's feet are challenged the more balanced, mobile and resilient they will be.

Ideally, your toddler needs lots of practice in different environments, and those on your doorstep are a perfect training ground. It is our responsibility as parents and carers to provide a variety of stimulation and opportunities.

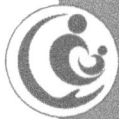

HOW TO INCREASE YOUR INFANT'S SENSORY INPUT AT THE FEET

At home
- Make your home a 'shoe-free' zone – you can control your environment at home so it should be safe to be inside and outside barefoot (weather/critter dependent).

Getting outdoors
- Back/front yard grass areas, pavement, sand pits and paddling pools all provide stimulation for the growing foot and a variety of movement opportunities.
- Go for walks.

- Take a trip to the beach and explore rocky foreshores, sand, seaweed and water.
- Explore inland forests, woods, and grasslands with soil, leaves, sticks, grass and mud.
- Local playgrounds and grassy areas can provide stimulation and space for the young feet to practice and explore.
- Be barefoot whenever possible.

Allow extra time for your toddler to walk places, with your help, rather than putting them in their stroller. I know it takes longer and more energy to walk with a toddler, but seeing the world from their level and eyes makes up for it. I recall having to stop and discuss snails in much more depth than I ever had with Nick one day. And then you just have to get creative when they start grizzling and are tired. Tell them cracks in the pavement emit energy, smelling flowers gives them super powers – anything to distract them. Although remember they may also really be tired so have the stroller ready or give them a piggy-back. Building tolerance for walking is important, so slowly increase time and distance.

Keep in mind though that the outdoors may present hazards depending on where you live so use footwear as necessary. Growing up in New Zealand, it was totally safe to play in long grass and in the bush, but my Australian family would think twice!

Baby walkers

Whilst it may be tempting to speed up your infant's journey to independent walking using devices such as baby walkers, these do not allow for natural exploration of their body and movement, nor do they help build strength and adaptability. This is similar to being propped up to sit.

Baby walkers have been banned entirely in Canada and their use strongly discouraged by medical associations in other countries due to the high number of injuries babies sustain while using them.

There are also harnesses you can put your infant in and trolleys they can push, all with amazing marketing statements and promises. I'd suggest saving your money and allowing your infant to follow their own inbuilt process for development.

Nature vs nurture

As a Structural Integration practitioner (someone who focuses on posture) I am intrigued by how people of all ages stand and move.

It is clear that infants do not copy their parents or siblings in their efforts to roll, crawl, squat or cruise, as these behaviours are not usually being modelled at the time of learning. They innately know what to do and how to do it through built-in reflexes, along with practice, trial and error, encouragement and sometimes surprise. I do wonder though when it comes to walking how much of what they observe in the adults around they take in and copy, thinking it's the right way. Next time you see a family walking down the road observe the similarities in their walking.

My friend Katja Bartsch, a fellow Structural Integration practitioner, yoga teacher, and sports science graduate, shared her story with me:

'We are all born with the ability to find an upright body posture with ease. We lose the ease in our posture mainly because we start copying and imitating at an early age. A small example from my own family: when my son started to run, he always held one arm close to his body (without swinging it along), the other arm flew through the air swinging vigorously back and forth. I could not understand why he was doing this and was quite puzzled by it. As a 'professional body observer', I watched his movement pattern with great interest. Finally, it became clear to me: we jog a lot.

Back then his dad pushed the stroller with one hand while the other arm took extra swing when he was running. So, my son always saw dad running with only one arm, the other arm was 'frozen'. Once we realised this, we made sure our little one had plenty of opportunity to observe the both of us running with both arms swinging along our sides and he eventually started to swing both of his arms, too.

However, it is usually not that clear. Children orient themselves in the smallest posture and movement patterns to the people they have in their immediate environment.'

Moral of the story: take some time to check out and address any of your own postural habits or compensations that perhaps are not serving you (i.e., if you have pain, discomfort or limited movement) to break the cycle of negative impacting patterns being passed on. This will also enable you to keep up with your infant as they grow, while helping your own feet and posture.

CHAPTER 8

FINDING THEIR FEET: WALKING

SO MUCH JOY IS INVESTED IN THOSE FIRST FEW STEPS BUT FEW of us understand the importance of all that development into mature, confident walking.

The journey to 'finding their feet' for your toddler begins with head control and the ability to hold and move their oversized skull (relative to their body) in gravity.

Time on the floor brings the early movements of flexion and extension and the development of their spinal curves, your toddler becoming stronger in the spinal and abdominal regions as ribs and pelvis learn to oppose each other. On their back they first find their feet, a new toy to play with (IMAGE 8.1).

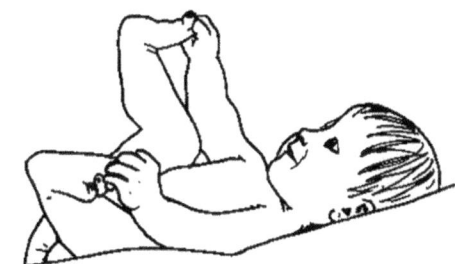

IMAGE 8.1: Feet are a great toy so don't hide them away.

Reaching for objects while lying on their tummy creates a side bending action, again causing opposition through their body. Patterns of lengthening and shortening change their body shape as they explore. On the floor weight is distributed broadly through their body.

Safe on the floor with no fear of falling, flexion and extension drives rotation and their first whole body movement to change position begins as they learn to roll. Their spine twists and a cascade of movement flows up and down their body.

As their overall strength increases your toddler rises up on all fours, rocks for a while and then tentatively begins contralateral movement of the limbs as they crawl forwards, or backwards. As one arm and the opposite leg moves forward, their small body also bends sideways (side flexion) and in time their head moves independently as they watch and look around. Crawling reduces their base of support to the four limbs, to three, then two when moving and they play here in gravity.

Moving in and out of sitting requires more flexion and extension, side movements, shifting their weight and rotations. Your toddler needs strength to push and lift their upper body into the vertical position whilst having a solid base of support with their bottom, legs and feet, propped at first by their arms.

They find their knees are useful props as they aim for higher. As they learn to stand, they reduce their base of support to just their tiny, underdeveloped flat feet, with all their weight being balanced between them. All the practice of flexing and extending, moving the head, ribs and pelvis has come together and they explore their centre of balance, helped of course by their puppeteer and various bodily systems (vestibular, sensory, motor). Your toddler's feet get their first experience of full pressure as they meet the ground, changing pressure (left to right, forward and back) as their body sways above. Continuous messages are sent from the feet to the brain, and tissue such as the plantar fascia develop for support.

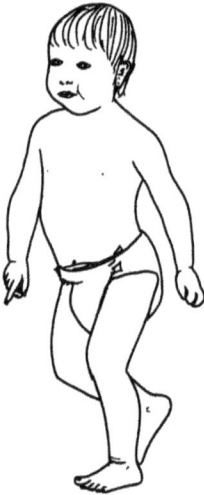

IMAGE 8.2: 80% of walking is spent standing, balancing and moving forward on one leg.

Lifting one foot and placing it a bit further afield, your toddler starts cruising around furniture, with hands providing extra support as their base of support reduces to one foot as they step to the left or right. The messages between their feet and brain adjust the tensioning cables in their feet and around their body as they manoeuvre and explore this new upright world.

As their confidence, awareness and strength grows, your toddler will eventually take their first steps forwards. All this requires balance, coordination and sensory input from the feet.

Walking requires the ability to shift their weight and stand on one leg (IMAGE 8.2) and their body to coordinate movement in the many directions teetering on their tripod: forwards, backwards, side-to-side, bending, tilting and rotating. All these movements are the collection of experiences provided by reflexes and previous milestones.

FORWARD MOTION

With the opportunity to practice, your toddler will become more confident and no doubt more adventurous on their two feet. So how do they actually move forward?

Think about the efficiency of a rubber band. You stretch it to fire it and it then goes back to its resting length. In the body we have something similar; it's called the 'stretch-shortening cycle'.[26] Your toddler has been toning theirs as they progressed through the milestones and reflex responses.

It can also be referred to as 'pre-tensioning', which is the controlled lengthening (an eccentric contraction) of the myofascia around a joint or along a line of action. This is the body's energy-saving tool for reducing effort required. Why would you use your whole arm to throw a rubber band at someone when stretching it with just your fingers and letting it fire across the room is much more effective? (I'm sure we've all got that wee evil streak in us sometimes.)

Pre-tensioning is a whole-body experience with multiple rubber bands lengthening at once. One good example of this is when you throw a ball, you take your arm backwards to pre-tension the tissue from the front of your shoulder down to your hip, and that helps you throw the ball with more power. Add a rotation to your ribs and more wind up, and this will result in even more power.

This efficiency will take some time to develop, with their gait not fully maturing until the age of eight. All this pre-tensioning happens in 3D because as your toddler walks, every part of their body has to change

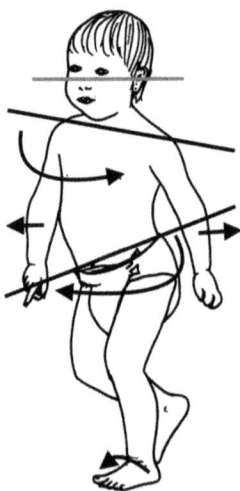

IMAGE 8.3: Walking requires movement in multiple planes, some are shown here, but there's so much more I assure you!

position, ribs tilt and rotate, the pelvis tilts and rotates, the curves of the spine change, the spine bends to the side in response to the ribs and pelvis and so on. The human body is complex, and so is walking!

As your toddler's walking gets better their head control improves. Their body will move under their head in ALL directions (planes of motion) and responding to the placement of their feet. The neck and vestibular system coordinate the balance of the head like the gimble used for mobile phones and camera videos. This is an intricate and highly tuned system, as are the feet (IMAGE 8.3).

FEET WERE MADE FOR WALKING: PRONATION AND SUPINATION

We will finish this chapter by heading back down to the feet, looking at the role they have to play in their position between the body and the ground.

'Pronation' and 'supination' are common terms for describing the collective movement of all parts of the foot in mature walking. Inside your toddler's feet these events will be starting to happen and patterns laid down.

Pronation (think flat foot) is when the arches of the foot drop down towards the ground in response to an increase of weight and forward motion over the foot. When the off-centred heel hits the ground, it creates a domino effect down through the foot bones, opening the joints on the sole side and creating a wider, longer and flatter looking foot. In response to the bones moving and joints opening, tissues will lengthen. Pronation is the stretched rubber band scenario under the foot, that can only respond by shortening. The leg bones have to follow the ankle bone (talus) so end up rotating inwards, lengthening and tensioning other tissues (rubber bands) **(IMAGE 8.4)**.

The opposite to a flat, pronated foot is a supinated one, with supination being the foot's journey from being flat (pronated) to twisted up on toes (supinated). The leg responds by rotating outwards, and the foot becomes twisted with a curved arch and rigid with the joints in the arch closing. This final position provides stability for the foot to act like a catapult to help propel us forward from the big toe.

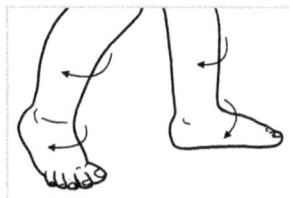

IMAGE 8.4: The unique shape of the foot bones creates movement in the foot, creating movement up the body. If the feet don't move, moving becomes an effort.

You could say that pronation is the sole of the foot opening, supination is it closing and in the middle is your toddler's tripod of support. Within these two actions each bone and joint in the foot (and the rest of the body) will travel through each of the planes of motion – but that is way too much information for this book!

You won't necessarily see these movements in your toddler as their cute fat pad may hide what is happening until they are at least five.

The movement back and forth between pronation and supination, lengthening and shortening of the foot, helps it manage the forces we experience. Pronation helps absorb and dissipate impact forces and the rigid lever position of supination creates a solid platform to release energy used for the forward swing of the leg. The foot's adaptability is all down to its unique architecture, an arrangement that is partly created by movement as we develop in utero and in our early years. The forces experienced by the foot help form and shape its bones and strengthen the soft tissues.

Hopefully you can see the feet need to be free as they grow. Free to go from flat to twisted with no fancy arch supports or stiff soles of shoes stopping them.

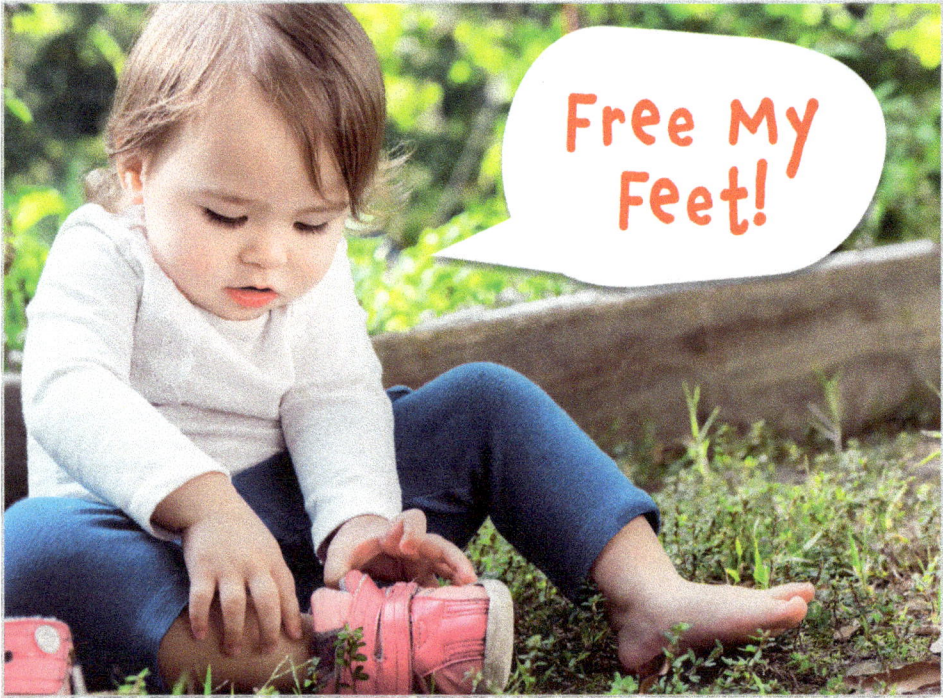

IMAGE 8.5: Free their feet!

BEYOND WALKING

Your toddler will spend the next eight or so years mastering walking and discovering the joys of running, jumping, skipping, more climbing and other movements for pleasure.

The home environment can provide much of the necessary stimulation and space for these activities but the great outdoors will challenge them more. There are many books with brilliant ideas such as:

- *Balanced and Barefoot* by Angela J. Hanscom
- *Grow Wild* by Katy Bowman
- *Last Child in the Woods* by Richard Louv

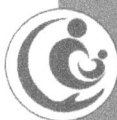

IDEAS FOR THE ACTIVE, MOBILE TODDLER

- Simple obstacle courses providing a mix of climbing, crawling and jumping.
- Balance beams on the ground (a simple length of 3"/8 cm × 2"/6 cm wood), raising them with bricks as their confidence grows.
- Writing with their feet.
- Statues game, challenge them more with one-legged statues.
- Squatting to do puzzles – remove toddler chairs.
- Free dance time, turn up the music and join them.
- Balance bikes.
- Parent climb – with your toddler facing you, hold their hands and have them walk up your legs and then flip over.
- Help them do hand/head stands, provide pillows for crash mats.
- Games like hopscotch and leap frog.
- Climbing trees, slopes and walls.
- Crab walking, toe-walking, moving backwards.
- Have them help you carry the shopping, or help in the garden.

The list really is endless; think about what you did as a child.

Venues such as trampoline parks and playgyms can give you a break whilst challenging your child's abilities and continue the all-important inner growth for balance, mobility and confidence.

Formal activities such as gymnastics, swimming, dance and athletics also offer different benefits, from maintaining flexibility and mobility, to helping with balance and coordination. Remember that play is how children learn best so until they show an interest to 'train' in an activity, as the saying goes, 'let kids be kids'.

The benefits of physical activity go beyond the development of their body. During the first three years your toddler's brain is developing rapidly, doubling in size during their first year. Their brain is hungry for and needs stimulation for all those neural connections. A wide range of experiences will lay the foundations for their overall health and well-being. And talking of foundations, back to their feet ...

CHAPTER 9

THE CASE FOR GOING BAREFOOT

I WAS AT OUR LOCAL PLAYGROUND 'DOING RESEARCH' – pretending to read a book whilst enjoying the sun.

I observed a young boy climbing up the slide and then a younger female friend try the same, unsuccessfully. Then the boy claimed he had great grip on his shoes, which must be why he could do it and she couldn't. She was wearing trainers. The mother of the girl, overhearing the conversation and seeing the frustration, said that next time she could wear her sandals for better grip.

I so desperately wanted to go over and whisper in the girl's ear, 'Take your shoes off.'

Whilst I don't make a habit of stalking young children in playgrounds, on another day I observed young twins running around in yellow rubber boots. The sun was out, but they were prepared for the regular winter rains. They started to climb the bars on the round jungle gym and really struggled with getting a good foot placement to step up. How could they feel the bar through the sole of the boots? Wouldn't they be safer without boots so they could feel the bar, and get a good grip before heading higher? Or was this a ploy by the parent to keep them within arm's reach?

SKIN

Take a close look at your infant's soles. You'll notice there are no hairs as soles and palms have what's called 'glabrous' skin. This is a thick layer of skin swimming with thousands of nerve endings, and is considered a major organ for sensing the external environment.[27]

Now take a closer look and you will see ridges or lines that make that cute, unique footprint (IMAGE 9.1). Beyond predicting love and life expectancy (according to some), the undulating surface allows for movement and increases the surface area of their foot, thus increasing their ability to grip and twist, and for the foot to expand.

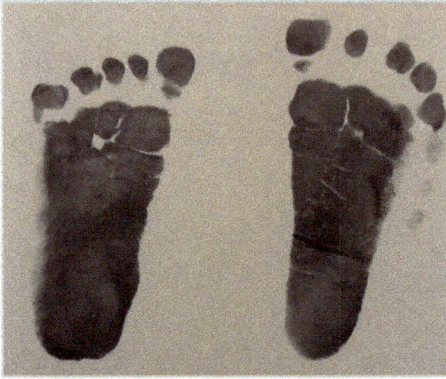

IMAGE 9.1: Evy's foot print (aged five months). (Photo: A Bennett)

Have you ever thought about why feet get all wrinkly after a long bath or soak in the hot tub? There's one popular theory about absorbing water and the outer layer of our skin swelling, but a more likely reason is thanks to our self-regulating body and the spontaneous reflex to increase our surface area for gripping when wet. You might have seen racing cars changing their tyres to suit the conditions, slicks for dry weather and rain (anti-hydroplaning) ones for the wet. How amazing is our body that it does it automatically, with no need to change feet. (Care still needs to be taken when there is water on the kitchen or bathroom floor.)

The skin itself is also an amazing barrier, designed to protect. So, if you are worried about dirt and the germs or disease your infant's bare foot could be exposed to, stop a moment and think about the environment created in the shoe. With more sweat glands in the feet than anywhere else on your body, there is more risk of fungal and bacterial infections from wearing shoes (just ask any mum of a teenage son!). You're also more likely to get sick from hand–mouth contact. Think about what kids touch in a day: playground equipment, rails, toilets. And given the world's recent pandemic, we are all now experts on hand hygiene.

My dear friend Peggy Dawson, founder of the New Zealand chapter of the International Association of Infant Massage and who taught me infant massage years ago, shared some of her story:

'In my day [the late 1940s] we went barefoot to school and throughout the school holidays. It wasn't until I went to university

in Wellington and was in Woburn Hostels in the Hutt, I remember our Matron telling me not to go barefoot because dogs peed and men spat on the pavements, which made me begin to wear shoes more often. I saw a video recently of a Maori woman telling her nieces and nephews to take off their shoes because they will get sick. It was unhealthy to wear shoes, and our feet should be connected to the earth. It was much healthier to go bare feet. I love the feel of my bare feet on wet lawn. Of course English people were completely horrified to see me walk bare foot down the street when we lived in West Byfleet, Surrey.'

THE BENEFITS OF GOING BAREFOOT

Apart from horses and the occasional dog, we are the only mammal that's decided to put something on our feet. Shoes have been around forever it would seem so why would we question their design or even existence?

In an attempt to further support my mission of preventing future failing feet I went in search of research. What is science saying about going barefoot and about wearing footwear?

FOOTWEAR RESEARCH

There is limited information on the impact of infants wearing shoes, and even those who have tried have found that a science lab is far from an infants' natural environment, and getting them to cooperate is a challenge.

From research on older children, we can draw some conclusions, hypothesise, overlay our new knowledge and make more informed decisions.

The discussion on the impact of the shoe of the foot is nothing new. In 1905, Phil Hoffman, MD, studied the feet of 186 Philippine and Central African people attending the 1904 Louisiana Purchase Exposition, a world fair in USA.[28] He used a wide range of measures – techniques which would be considered archaic today – such as foot prints on smoked paper and plaster of Paris moulding. He compared those habitually barefoot to those who wore shoes.

Dr Hoffman's relevant findings on going barefoot

- When sitting, the toe bones of a barefoot person lined up with the metatarsals and when standing, the toes separated to give a wide base of support.
- The sole of the foot was thick, tough, pliable and free from calluses.
- The big toe provided leverage.

Dr Hoffman's observations on people who wore shoes

- High heels resulted in weight shifting to forefoot, and tight calves.
- Feet were narrow with no spread of toes.
- A reduced range of motion in ankle and joints of foot.

In his concluding report to the Association of Orthopedic Surgeons, he suggested that society and manufacturers regulate the shape and style of shoes, believing that over time the wearer gets used to the compressed feeling and ceases to be aware of any ill fit. Whilst Hoffman's study focused on the adult population, we can consider the results as the impact of being barefoot or not, through life.

A century on, podiatrist Dr William A. Rossi authored many articles and several books on feet, confirming and advancing Hoffman's earlier findings on the impacts of wearing shoes. In one article, he noted:

'It took four million years to develop our unique human foot and our consequent distinctive form of gait ... in only a few thousand

years, and with one carelessly designed instrument, our shoes, we have warped the pure anatomical form of human gait, obstructing its engineering efficiency, afflicting it with strains and stresses and denying it its natural grace of form and ease of movement head to foot.'[29]

One of his articles, published in 2005, has always stood out to me: 'Children's Footwear: Launching Site for Adult Foot Ills.'[30] A great title, and potentially true. The subheadline of the article notes that it's 'time to advocate shoelessness for kids' – and that is a sentiment I definitely agree with.

PAEDIATRIC FOOTWEAR

In 2010 the *Guardian* (UK) newspaper featured an article titled 'Why Barefoot Is Best for Children'.[31] Tracy Bryne, a mother and paediatric podiatrist, was interviewed and had these key messages:

'Toddlers keep their heads up more when they are walking barefoot as they get feedback from the ground. Walking barefoot develops muscles and ligaments of the foot, increases the strength of the foot's arch, improves proprioception and contributes to good posture. The more parents know about the structure of children's feet, the more we can prevent footwear-related damage being done.'

I contacted her to see how education of parents was going ten years later. Her response was 'Sadly, there is a real lack of information and education on this subject.' My response – 'Best I do something about that then!'

In 2018 the Journal of Foot and Ankle Research[32] editorial stated that 'paediatric footwear is an aspect that is under investigation in relation to the perceived and potential effects on the development of the foot over time' and that appropriate footwear is vital for healthy feet. A narrative review in the same journal[33] found that there was more understanding needed of the interaction between the child's foot and shoe, and that there was a lack of evidence and data to support any decision about whether shoes were better or not for the developing foot.

We need to look at the bigger picture: the impact of footwear on the growing foot and its relationship and influence on the rest of the body, and on how we stand and move. So I kept digging ...

A review of eleven studies in 2011 by researchers at the University of Sydney,[34] and a similar review by researchers in Melbourne, Australia, in 2019,[35] came to the overall conclusion that shoes affect gait in the following two ways:

- stride length and speed of walk increased due to extra length of leg (from height of shoe sole) and weight from shoe
- restrictions in foot motion from wearing shoes resulted in increased hip and knee movement.

One article I found really interesting was one that found cushioned heels result in a heavier, harder heel strike, almost as if the heel was searching for the impact to trigger the foot's reaction for walking.[36] It makes sense if you think about the foot being a sensory connection to the ground. Another potential reason for your infant to be unshod as they grow and develop – cushioned heels can be acting like a dampener.

Other studies[37] on children walking in footwear with a heel, narrow and raised toe box with a rigid sole found the following:

- the heavier the shoe, the more energy required
- increased muscle use meant increased oxygen consumption

- decreased muscle activity in the foot
- changes in lower limb kinetics (reactions)
- less capacity to store elastic energy in the Achilles tendon
- reduced shock absorption
- reduction in toe extension by 30–45 degrees
- overall changed biomechanics of the foot.

If footwear changes the way your infant learns to walk, requires more energy and oxygen, alters your infant's position in space and potentially cause damage to the foot, why do we all keep buying them?

MYTHS AND MARKETING

In his 2002 article, Rossi[38] alluded to the role of marketing of shoes, with manufacturers claiming that shoes were 'healthy for child foot development' and 'shoes will help your child walk properly', which are unsubstantiated claims.

Has anything changed? Do we ever pause and question retailers?

Or do we assume, surely if they are selling the product, it must be okay for us? Most parents I speak with use a popular shoe company simply because everyone else does; no one thinks to question whether the footwear is appropriate or not. I definitely didn't when my boys were little.

There are also various myths floating around when it comes to buying footwear for children's young feet; myths such as allowing room to grow, a snug fit and needing support for arch, ankle and heel. Let's unpack some of those myths based on what we now know.

- 'Buying shoes to grow in to.' NO! Shoes are designed to bend in line with toes bending; a mis-match with a longer shoe will affect foot biomechanics.

- A 'snug fit' in the midfoot is NOT necessarily best as it may stop the foot's ability to move and it's need to spread.
- Doing the shoe up too tightly may restrict blood flow, arteries and nerves, along with stopping movement.
- 'Support for the arch, ankle and heel' DOES NOT allow for natural free movement of tissues and bones (pronation/supination), and the growth of a strong structure.

Only in understanding the foot itself can we dispel these myths and create a new social norm where barefoot, or foot-like footwear is accepted because it is healthier for your child growing up.

In clinical practice, I see a wide range of foot ailments in adults attached to bodies with other symptoms and conditions, a common one being back pain. The 'other' is where treatment used to start, but these days nine times out of ten I start at the feet! And many of my clients have no idea about the importance of their feet.

One could argue that it is the shoes we wear as adults that do the damage, but hopefully you can see that during the early years, when the foot is growing, there is greater potential for damage and it may be where it all starts. Issues can lie dormant like a volcano for years. What we put on our infant's feet may come back to haunt them in the future. And this is nothing new.

Today, the shelves are stocked and the internet littered with 'foot pain' solutions. Why? Have you ever thought about it? Not to mention all the various therapists and medical professionals trained to deal with aches and pains. As the saying goes, prevention is better than cure. We can do better for our kids.

What do you want your baby's feet to look like in twenty or thirty years?

THE PLASTIC FOOT

Back in 1905, Hoffman[39] described the foot as very plastic, able to be moulded to any shape. Humans are both plastic and elastic (our rubber bands). We are elastic in the sense that we are always changing shape with movement and breath returning to our centre, our place of rest, by our elastic nature. The elastic properties of fascia inside us allow for this movement, as well as absorbing stress and withstanding strain. Plasticity, on the other hand (or foot), is about changing, morphing our shape slowly over time due to external influences, habits and patterning.

One example of how the body can be moulded is the tradition of foot binding in China, dating back to the 10th century. Deemed a status symbol of the elite, a girl's feet were bound within the lotus shoe, a practice that continued into the 1940s and even beyond despite being banned by the ruling party. At the age of five to six years, a girl's feet were bound tightly, after all the small toes were broken and folded. This process of break and bind would continue over the next two years with the end result being a 'beautiful' delicate foot described as being like the lotus flower. The actual result was a small, yet hugely deformed, restricted pair of feet (IMAGE 9.2). Ouch!

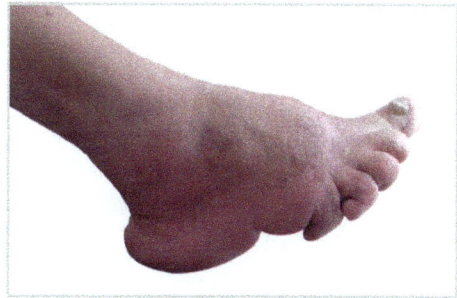

IMAGE 9.2: Foot binding, the result of an age-old tradition that only stopped in the 1940s.

One could consider practices like foot binding, wearing a corset, and neck, lip and ear stretching early forms of plastic or cosmetic surgery – not using a knife, but an external force applied over time. All, except perhaps the ear stretching, would have left the woman far from functioning normally (women seem to always be the ones affected by such cultural traditions).

If we place footwear on a continuum, the lotus shoe would be at one end with barefoot at the other, and the rest of shoes spread along the spectrum depending on their influence on the foot (and of course how long they are worn).

I passionately believe that children should go barefoot as much as possible up to the age of five, beyond if possible. For your child, playing and walking barefoot:

- allows for optimal sensory development
- improves spatial awareness, balance and posture
- enhances motor development and coordination
- provides greater foot strength, muscle activity and mobility
- reduces clumsiness and increases greater grip and stability
- allows for optimal growth and development
- is economical – bare feet cost nothing.

We could conclude that structural changes lead to functional changes. Poorly designed footwear has the potential to change both the structure and function of the foot, and therefore the body as everything is connected. When will footwear manufacturers consider the foot and function over fashion?

CHAPTER 10

THE EVOLUTION OF FOOTWEAR

HOW DID FASHION TRUMP FUNCTION?

In 3000 BC, Egyptians created sandals to protect their feet from the hot sand. The concept of the sandal was also adopted by other warmer regions around the world such as the Mexicans with their huaraches (native sandal), Japanese zori sandals were worn with traditional kimono and the Romans wore sandals laced up their legs.

Sandals were made from a wide range of natural plant materials including seaweed, bark, straw and wood. In New Zealand, paraerae (flax) and cabbage tree leaves were plaited and woven to provide protection. Most were not designed for daily use, let alone to stand the test of time, but traditions do live on in many cultures, if somewhat adapted such as the thong, flip-flop or jandal (Japanese sandal).

The sole of the original Roman sandal was made of cork with a leather upper. Animal skins were widely used as they were soft and pliable, able to be wrapped around the foot. Indigenous Australians used emu feathers on the soles of shoes to obscure their footprints as they travelled. The military Roman sandal was reinforced with hobnails that could also leave imprints of messages. Skins were also used to bind and cover injuries to the foot, and perhaps that was an 'ah-ha' moment that prevention is better than cure.

Protection was predominantly from the environment and weather. People in extreme cold climates such as those living close to the Arctic Circle opted not for a breezy sandal but a snug, enclosed boot made from animal fur and skins, in particular reindeer and seal. The Inuit would first use the seal skin to store seal fat then wild berries, both to impregnate the skin with oil to make it waterproof before turning it into a mukluk or kamik (long boot). The Japanese ashida (rain shoe) is fascinating. It's a shoe for the rain, but think wellington, gumboot, rubber boot, galoshes, etc., and you'd be wrong! They are raised wooden clog like a sandal with two slats under the sole that can be as high as 10 cm.

As footwear developed over time, it became more of a status and fashion symbol, welcoming high heels, stylish shapes, decorations, shoe linings (aka socks) and more. You may know King Henry VIII for his wives, but you may not know he wore a 'duckbill' style of shoe with broad toe (created for Charles VIII of France who had an extra toe). Eventually his daughter Queen Mary I outlawed them, which was a good thing as it made wearers waddle!

Jump forward a hundred years to Louis XIV of France, who took the Persian design of a practical high heel that secured a boot in a horse's stirrup and turned it into a fashion statement, often elaborately decorated with depictions of battle scenes. Furthermore he made red heels a sign of aristocracy; only those in favour with the royals could wear them!

For many years shoes were uniform, and one shape for both feet, with no differentiation between left or right (perhaps where 'my two left feet' arose from?). Women have worn platform shoes and heels over the centuries, but it wasn't until after World War II that they started getting more sophisticated and narrower.

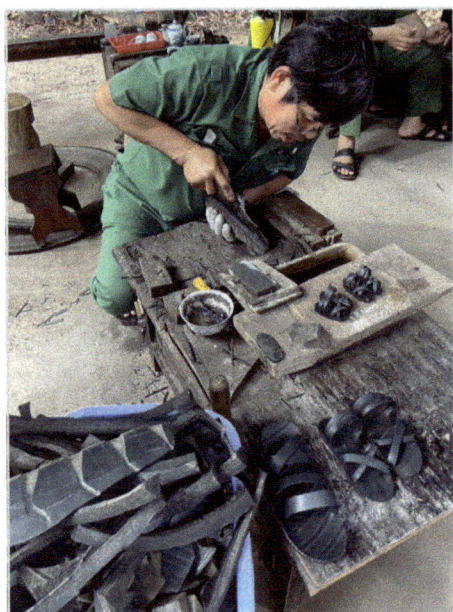

IMAGE 10.1: Vietcong sandal being made out of old tyres. (Photo: B Landels)

When in Vietnam, I visited the Cu Chi Tunnels, a 121 km underground network just outside Ho Chi Minh City. Here I observed the making of Vietcong sandals from old tyres (IMAGE 10.1). Cheap to make and repair, they were not only worn for hygiene in the hot humidity (think of the Americans in their boots, eeew) but the soldiers could trick the enemy by turning the shoes around and make like the footprints (tread) were going the other way.

Fast forward to today and I wonder if the likes of Richard Branson, Elon Musk and Alicia Keys can be as influential as the royals of the past. They, amongst others are all choosing to live 'shoe optional' lifestyles.

SOCKS

The other footwear I should mention is the sock. They were deemed 'lightweight shoes' and made originally from leather or animal hair in 8th century BC. Over the centuries they have been knitted and sewn from many different fabrics. It was around the Middle Ages that they became more of an accessory rather than necessity for warmth and protection. Like the shoe they eventually became a fashion accessory and status symbol. And like the multitude of shoes for different looks and activities, you can get a sock for just about anything you do too these days, and in almost any colour, pattern or material, with each design having proven features such as cushioning or breathability.

INFANT FOOTWEAR HISTORY

The history of infants' footwear is less documented. One could presume that infants were unshod or that they wore a smaller version of the adult form. In ancient Greece, to be 'sandaled' was the rite of passage for a seven-year-old boy as they started school and for girls it was when they married. In Europe, they swaddled (tightly wrapping) limbs of newborns in the early 18th century, and the 19th century has records of the knitted baby bootie. Early shoes were designed with practicality in mind, and over time styles emerged made of leather with rounded toe, low heels, a mix of lace-up, buckles or slip-on, some with zippers or elastic sides.

In 1968, the Puma shoe company introduced velcro for adult performance shoes, with other sports shoe companies following suit, which soon impacted shoe fastening options for everyone – including infants. There are more velcro infant shoes on the market now than lace-up. 'A Parent's Guide to Buying Toddler Shoes', an online guide published in the Huffington Post, provides tips such as: 'If your toddler's a wriggler, velcro is the easiest to do up; but if they love pulling socks and shoes off, then buckles or laces may be better to outwit them.'[40] Velcro is a godsend for parents, and a timesaver, but you now need the activity book with shoelaces in more than ever to teach the fine motor skills for tying bows.

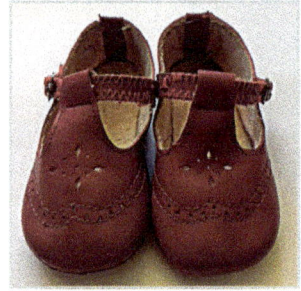

IMAGE 10.2: Talking of history – these were my first ever shoes, dating back to the early 1970s.
(Photo: C Landels)

And for me there is the question of why do shoes and socks get pulled off by infants wearing them? What are infants trying to tell us?

CHAPTER 11

WHAT IS THE BEST FOOTWEAR FOR CHILDREN?

WE KNOW BEING BAREFOOT IS BEST FOR LEARNING, EXPLORING and most importantly moving. But there may be times when it is not practical or safe, and – given the concrete jungle most of us live in – not comfortable. Or there may be occasions when your infant has to wear something on their tootsies to conform to society's rules or expectations, or you just prefer them to.

Go to any major infant shoe supplier (in person or online) and you will find hundreds of shoes and socks for every size, and different ones for each stage of development (for example, crawlers, cruisers, pre-walkers), which can add to your confusion. I even found you could buy knee pads for the crawling stage. Needless to say, I was gobsmacked. You might need them if you're going to take up crawling again but your infant definitely doesn't need them!

With so many different types of footwear available, how does one make a decision on what is best for the growing foot? There is limited, but promising, research available. In 2020, a small study (thirteen toddlers with an average age of 13.3 months) in Melbourne, Australia looked at whether soft-soled footwear such as the Bobux XPLORER would affect gait.[41] Each of these shoes only weighs 30 grams and the upper is made of soft leather. They compared barefoot walking with the soft-soled footwear and found that there was minimal difference in gait (IMAGE 11.1).

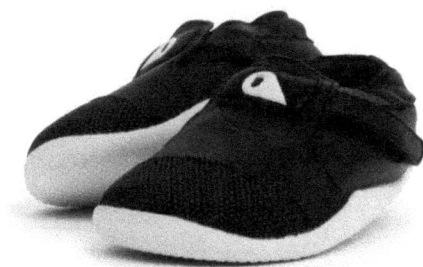

IMAGE 11.1: Bobux Xplorer Black Origin shoe used in the research.

This research is promising and supports the design for a shoe that is more closely aligned with the infant foot, and one that serves the basic need of the foot, which is protection. I do wonder if there will come a time when footwear replicating the human foot is just common sense and we don't need to prove anything! Ideal footwear for your infant's growing feet is:

- foot-shaped
- light
- flexible
- flat
- less is best, think minimal.

MINIMAL SHOES

In the 1990s, the 'barefoot', or minimalistic, shoe made a comeback. Remember, historically, footwear was mostly for protection. A minimalistic shoe provides protection whilst allowing the foot to function closer to what a bare foot does. More foot-like than shoe-like!

'If we start our kids out by wearing minimalistic shoes, there will be no adaptation that's needed as adults and I believe that this could be one piece of the holy grail in reducing musculoskeletal injuries in adults.' **DR IRENE DAVIS, PROFESSOR AT HARVARD MEDICAL SCHOOL**[42]

Let's look at some minimal infant shoes, their structure and what benefits they give the young developing foot.

In 1985, in Oregon, USA, the Softstar shoe company was born when founder Tim Oliver was unable to find minimal shoes for his baby girl. In 1991, in a New Zealand garage, Bobux created their first 'Soft Sole' minimal shoe. The first Inch Blue shoe was made at a kitchen table in Wales, UK, in 1998 when a mum spotted a gap in the local market for colourful, functional baby's shoes. And down in Melbourne, a New Zealand mum teamed up with an Australian mum to put the 'fun' back in functional children's footwear with PaperKrane in 2012.

I love the fact that many creations of shoes for small feet came from individuals and families looking for a solution for their own loved ones.

Please be assured there are other manufacturers and retailers of suitable minimal footwear for your infant. Shop around and keep in mind – less is best. Or head to my website for a list.

Anatomy of a shoe

The anatomy of a minimal shoe is similar to the traditional shoe, sort of. Think army tank versus Formula One racing car, or elephant versus leopard! There are so many parts of the 'traditional' shoe, and they vary from shoe to shoe, from the tongue and moustache to foxing and vamps. Let's just focus on a simple shoe for your baby. The Bobux company sums it up beautifully: when it comes to design, the only five features of a shoe that matter are flexibility, adjustability, breathability, weight, and fit (IMAGE 11.2).

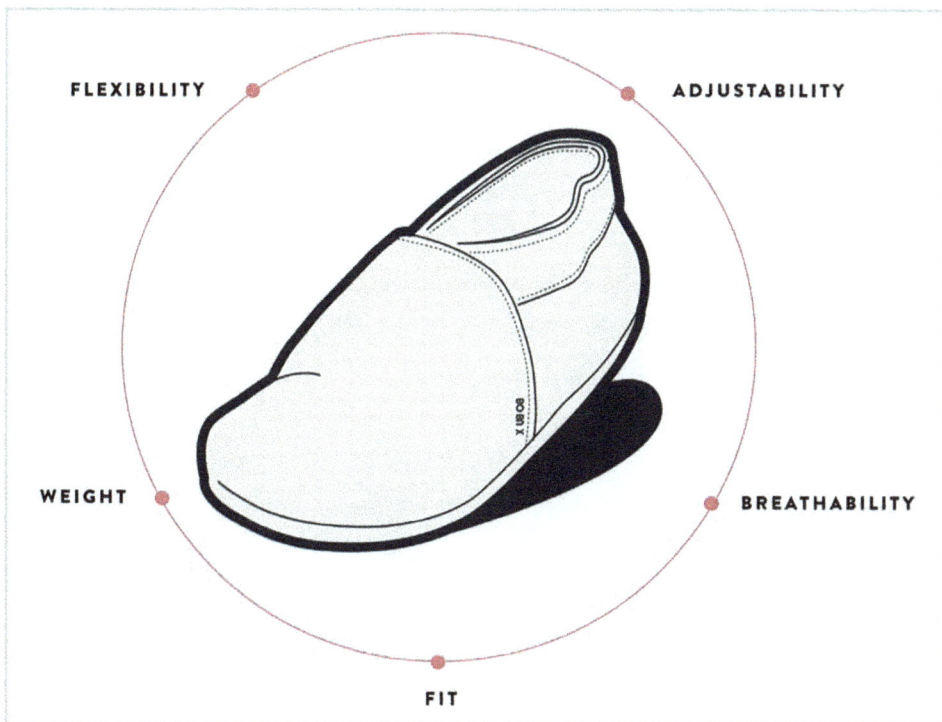

FLEXIBILITY   ADJUSTABILITY

WEIGHT   BREATHABILITY

FIT

IMAGE 11.2: Bobux (NZ) shoe design.

The last is first

A shoe is made from the inside out, around a mould called a 'last'. This determines the various dimensions of a shoe: the height of the uppers along with the length and width, particularly of the toe box, and the height of the toe spring. Those in the business of making minimal shoes, especially for little feet, have clearly done their research into how feet naturally move and function, and the foot's impact on posture. I am not sure what feet other manufacturers are looking at!

You don't have to be a engineer to know that a wide base of support is better than narrow. Minimal shoes are much wider in the forefoot than traditional shoes and take a little to get used to in terms of look but once we have the majority of children wearing them, they will become the norm.

Toe box and spring for foot function

The toe box and spring should be wide and flat. Wide to accommodate the spread of your infant's forefoot as we have already explored, and flat because toes don't stick up, do they? If toes are held in a raised position, this can increase the strain on the plantar fascia (bottom of foot), challenging and straining the base of support and balance. If we go back to our rubber band analogy, imagine holding the rubber band taut for a couple of hours; you'd get tired. In a raised, rigid toe box, the toes are held upwards and tissues already partially pretensioned, so there is less elastic range available, less efficiency, the foot will tire easily and timing will be affected.

If we also consider the bones, remember your infant's forefoot is developed ahead of their hindfoot, with the midfoot maturing last. It is therefore important that there is space and flatness for movement providing the best environment for the other bones to move and develop within (IMAGE 11.3).

Footwear that allows the toes to rest in 'neutral' and expand with movement, provide the best environment for optimal, efficient movement and development of the infant foot.

I suspect 'bunion' may come to mind for some of you when you see a narrow toe box (IMAGE 11.3) – hold on until Chapter 12.

The sense-able sole

A thin sole provides both flexibility and sense-ability (IMAGES 11.4 & 11.5).

The more supportive, formed and rigid the sole of a shoe, the weaker and less functional your infant's foot will become over time.[43]

IMAGE 11.3: Squashed or unsquashed? An inside view of what may happening to toes. (Photo: @barfussfreaks)

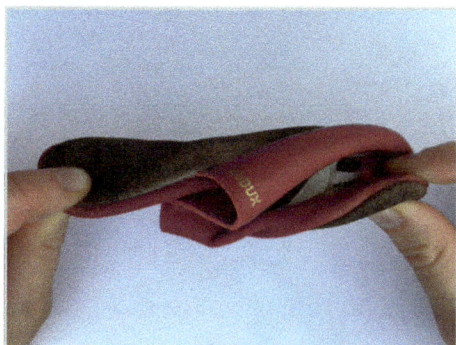

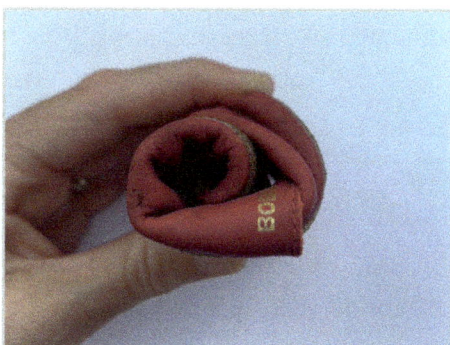

Your infant's toes need to bend to push forward in walking and also to get up on tip toes. These two actions require the big toe (the first metatarsophalngeal joint) to be able to bend between 40 and 90 degrees.[44] Now put a rigid sole under the foot and I'm sure you can imagine what will happen, or rather what will not. The big toe joint needs to be free to move, to stretch the elastic bands under the foot to help with propelling the body forward with the least amount of effort.

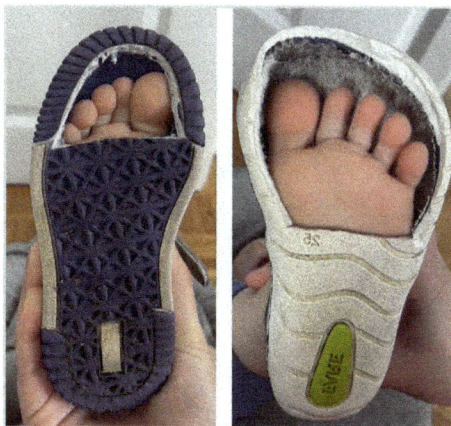

IMAGES 11.4 & 11.5: Bobux 'Soft Sole' shoes can be rolled and twisted allowing the foot flexibility and feeling. (Photo: B Landels)

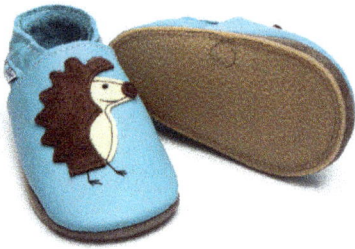

IMAGE 11.6: Inch Blue (UK) 'Gripz Spike' shoe with extra grip from a rubber sole added to their soft sole shoe.

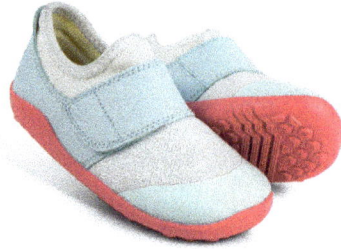

IMAGE 11.7: Bobux 'I-Walk Dimension II' shoe with great tread.

Pause for a moment and check out your own toe flexibility. Lift your toes, stand on tip toes, kneel with toes tucked under pointing forwards. How flexible and straight is your big toe?

Flexible footwear allows for full, efficient movement and the thinner the sole the better the sensitivity, proprioceptive awareness and adaptability to the ground below, though still not as good as a bare foot.

Once your infant is walking tread becomes important too, for both flexibility and grip. Simple grip like Inch Blue's 'Gripz' or Bobux's 'I-Walk Dimension II' are perfect (**IMAGES 11.6 & 11.7**). Even if you find a shoe that looks like it's got a good tread, if it doesn't tick the flexibility box then give them a miss. Both your infant's posture and gait have to adapt when they wear shoes with a thick, hard or spongy, often unbendable, sole.

The heel and its relationship to posture

When it comes to children, high heels are great for playing dress-up, and that's about it.

The 'drop' of a shoe is the difference in height between the heel and the forefoot. In a 'zero drop' shoe, there is no difference in this height, allowing your infant's feet to be in a similar position as if standing bare-foot, i.e., flat.

If we placed any footwear with raised heels (think wedge) under your infant's feet, their centre of mass would shift as they lean forward, changing their natural posture (IMAGE 11.8). They would either have to bend like a banana (lean back), or counterbalance by sticking their bum out behind and thrusting their upper body and head forward. Heels directly impact centre of balance. The flow on effect of this changes how they walk, as we saw in the research on page 119.

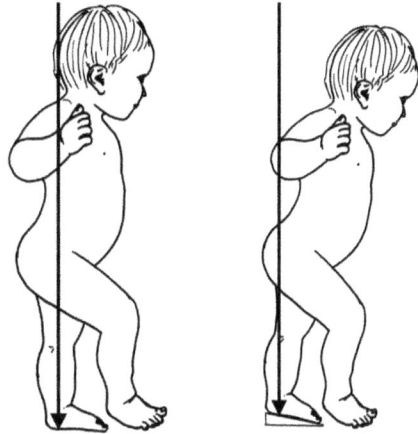

IMAGE 11.8: *Left*: Natural posture when standing or walking is centred and balanced. *Right*: Place a shoe on their foot that has a heel and they will have to adapt their posture so as not to fall forwards. Any shoe with a heel WILL affect their centre of balance, posture and change how they walk.

I was amazed to find a style of shoe for early walkers available for purchase that had a squeaky heel insert. Apparently, it was designed to encourage the child to learn how to heel strike when walking. While most children won't need any extra help developing a mature stepping pattern, and most certainly don't need the added height of a heel insert, it could give positive feedback to the habitual toe-walker and therefore act as encouragement to break the habit.

The upper fabric

We've talked about the toe box, sole and heel, so that leaves us the upper, tongue and heel cup to consider. A simple shoe is best: one made from natural breathable material, with minimal padding, that is adjustable, yet supportive and secure. High ankle support may limit ankle mobility, weakening myofascia and inhibiting proprioception. You want your infant to feel like they're not wearing anything and they don't have to grip with their toes to keep them on. It's important too that shoes are not fastened too tight as it is possible to constrict all the soft tissues, veins and nerves.

Put all of this together and you have a lightweight shoe that will allow your infant hours of running around without getting as tired, that helps ground their feet and stimulate them, whilst keeping their tootsies safe.

SOCKS

Socks are ideal for those pre-moving months and great for keeping toes warm, though I invite you to ask yourself why you think their feet are cold enough to require frequent covering. If it's not cold enough for you to consider wearing gloves on your hands, perhaps your baby's need for socks can be reconsidered.

Ensure any sock fits like the shoe: wide at the toes and not tight through the foot and ankle. Breathable, natural material is best. Whilst we want the sock to stay on, it is important they do not cause marks around the ankle. Think about the layers under the skin and how their bones have not fully hardened; any constant pressure will affect movement and flow of connective tissues, nerves and blood vessels. When teaching infant massage, this is one thing I look out for with new parents as they undress their baby. It can also happen in other areas of the body so check during nappy changing and bath time that there are no visible marks of where clothes have been too tight.

If your infant is wearing a sock/shoe combination, it is important that with the addition of the sock the shoe is not too tight.

Using milestones as a guide, let's look at some footwear options for your infant as they grow. This is a guide bringing together what we have just covered, using Bobux, Inch Blue, Softstar and PaperKrane as examples. They all have size guides available on their websites, with PaperKrane and Softstar also accounting for foot width.

PRE-MOVING FOOTWEAR

Throughout the book I have talked about how footwear serves the purpose to protect. So if you think about your baby and the early milestones before they start moving – what do you need to protect their feet from?

Socks and knitted booties are great to keep toes warm in cooler months and can provide protection from the sun. Don't let putting something on their feet be a default though as we regularly don't put anything on their wee hands. Often we assume our baby's feet are cold, especially if we ourselves have cold feet. Take a moment to feel both their hands and feet, then make a decision. If they feel the same, treat them the same. If you're going outside and it's cold and you'd put gloves on, then wrap up the feet too.

As mentioned, ensure socks and booties are not too tight around the ankles, and ensure plenty of space for your baby to wiggle their toes.

You might be wondering, does it really matter what they wear on their feet if they aren't moving and walking yet? Well, probably not, if it's for a short time. The foot is plastic and mouldable, remember, and you don't want to restrict their growth. So if you are heading out and about and wish to put shoes on, think foot before fashion! There are some really funky options available these days that tick all the boxes, including fashion.

Look for soft, light and flexible options such as Softstar's 'Moccasins' (IMAGE 11.9). Inch Blue and Bobux have 'Soft Soles', and PaperKrane 'Softi Soles'.

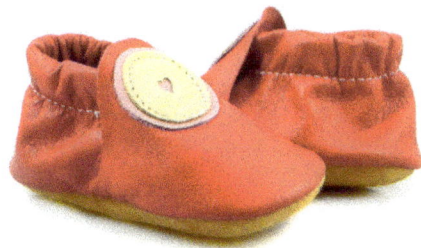

IMAGE 11.9: Softstar (USA) 'Moccasins' are light and flexible.

CRAWLING, STANDING, CLIMBING FOOTWEAR

As your infant begins crawling, they start to explore toe extension some more as they push their toes into the floor. So you need footwear that gives them both grip and flexibility. Being barefoot is best, followed by socks with grip pads.

If you're heading outdoors with your infant, then shoes with soft soles with their leather non-slip grip are one option. They will help protect your infant's toes more than socks and booties.

They are also designed for free mobility of both foot and ankle. This is important as your infant bends at the toes and ankle to achieve standing and climbing, whilst still providing a connection to the ground with the thin sole.

Footwear for cruising

As with all milestones, you need to think about what purpose the shoe is serving. At home there is often little need for protection. It is usually when you head to the urban jungle or playgrounds that you may want a little more protection for your nearly-toddler.

You may continue to have your infant in shoes like the Bobux Soft Soles, however the sole may take a hammering! With that in mind, Bobux designed a shoe range called Xplorer with a thin rubber sole to provide this extra protection, without losing the flexibility or adding any extra weight. Within this range, as with all, they have blended fashion with function as your infant is learning to walk. Inch Blue and PaperKrane (IMAGE 11.10) upgraded their soft soled options with rubber soles that still allow greater flexibility.

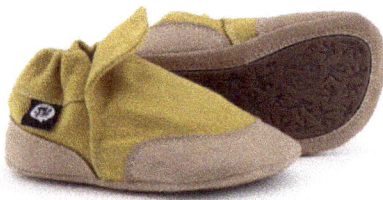

IMAGE 11.10: PaperKrane (AUST) 'Dijon.2' in their baby range provide a little more traction with customised rubber sole.

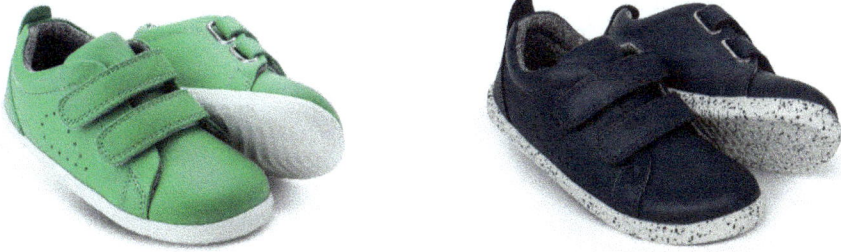

IMAGE 11.11: Bobux 'Step Up Emerald Grass Court' and 'I-Walk Navy Grass Court' shoe with horizontal tread to allow flexibility.

Walking footwear

Personally, I would stay with the softer style of shoe because the sole is thinner and more flexible, however for durability PaperKrane, SoftStar and Bobux have several lightweight designs for getting out and active; ideal for outdoors when the weather and environment prevent barefoot.

If you look closely at the Bobux Step Up range for novice walkers and the I-Walk range for toddlers, the soles have the extra feature of specially designed tread going across the soles for natural flexibility and grip **(IMAGE 11.11)**. I particularly like Bobux's open-toed sandals which allow the toes to be free and you can make sure they are not being squashed (not ideal for cold or wet weather, though). Remember your infant's foot will grow sneakily fast so check shoes regularly.

Think outside the box

Some brands of shoes designed for water activities meet the 'barefoot' minimal criteria and offer a more affordable option over other brands. They're designed to get wet and dry quickly so with socks would be ideal in winter for splashing in puddles.

Or if you are handy then grab some scraps of leather and make your baby's first pair yourself. I did! Search 'pattern for making soft sole shoe' on the internet and get started!

OTHER FOOTWEAR

There will be times as your child grows that you will need different footwear for activities or conditions. It's also likely that they will see different shoes advertised or worn by their friends, and they will nag you to buy the same ones.

It's ok for your child to wear other types of shoes, I would just suggest not all day or every day! Just as the need or purpose requires. Let's have a look at a few different ones:

Rainboots, wellingtons and gumboots

There are not many 'minimal' options available yet. The good thing is most rain boots are wider fitting and have no support inside but unfortunately they often have a raised heel. Try to find boots that have no heel raise if you can. Bobux offers the Paddington rainboot and several styles of other waterproof shoes, and Softstar sells the leather Phoenix boot that is lined with sheepskin and water resistant. If you find a shoe or boot that is ideal in shape and style, remember that if it is leather the waterproof quality can be increased by using a wax or waterproofer. Follow the suggestions for buying shoes on page 148 to ensure you are getting the right size, check sizing every couple of months, and limit the amount of time you have your toddler jumping around in them if they have a raised heel. And unless it's really cold, puddles are much better experienced barefoot!

Crocs

These seem to have become quite popular over recent years and given they are wide-fitting and light, they are not too bad on the spectrum of shoes. However, the thick spongey sole/heel would affect proprioception as well as heel strike, and most have a raised toe box.

Slippers

For slippers for inside and colder climates, you can't really go past any design with a soft sole like the Bobux Soft Soles.

Thongs, flip-flops and jandals

I have mixed feelings about this classic summer footwear. I grew up wearing them and loved them. They tick the box in terms of being spacious and most have a flexible sole, but are they good for our children's growing feet? I went hunting for research and found one study completed in Australia in 2013 and published in the *Journal of Foot and Ankle Research*.[45] This study concluded that there was minimal effect on walking, with some adaptations being a result of having to grip with the toes to hold the thong to the foot. I would suggest that short term use of such footwear, such as crossing the hot tarmac to the beach, is preferable to walking any real distance, such as to the shops or along the beach. Prolonged use would have ramifications on the function and condition of foot and lower leg myofascia. Any footwear that you have to grip with your toes surely will change your gait.

Ballet shoes

Having never done ballet myself I had to 'phone a friend' to check out first hand what a pair of ballet shoes were actually like.

With a soft leather sole, with satin or leather uppers held on to the foot with a ribbon or elastic they are designed with movement and flexibility in mind. With no support they are great for building foot strength. But that's where my positive review stops; once you enter the world of pointe shoes it surely can't end well.

WHAT TO LOOK FOR IN AN INFANT SHOE

- Thin, flexible sole for movement and sensitivity.
- Wide toe box so all toes can move and spread.
- Flat toe box for 'neutral' toes.
- Flat (zero drop) heel to allow optimal posture.

TIPS FOR SHOE SHOPPING WITH INFANTS

- Go prepared.
- Make a cardboard template. Draw and cut around your infant's feet with their toes spread, ideally standing so you get the widest spread of their foot and longest toe length. It would be best to do this after physical activity or the end of the day as kids' feet do change. This is a quick way to check which shoes match their foot size by inserting the template into the shoe. It will narrow down the number of shoes to try on, saving time and energy. Of course many child-specific retailers offer a measuring service which achieves the same thing.
- Allow time for your infant to walk, run and jump in them before you buy. A shoe should feel comfortable from the start. They shouldn't need 'wearing in', beside which your infant will outgrow them before that may happen!

If shopping online
- The cardboard template you made of your child's foot will help as you can easily measure length and width. Check that the size guide online reflects the size of the actual foot (not the sole of the shoe).
- Check their returns policy.

Re-use, recycle

Given that infants feet will normally out-grow a pair of shoes before they wear out, second-hand and hand-me-down minimal shoes should pose no problem as long as you check the size and fit properly. And given that most minimal shoes can be more expensive than 'normal' shoes, why not!

The older child (and yourself)

As your child grows the options for minimal shoes continue with the Vivobarefoot kids range in the United Kingdom, Wildling Shoes from Europe, and Xero Shoes in the United States. Most companies ship worldwide or have local stockists. It would be great if all shoe manufacturers came on board providing healthier options ... one day.

It just makes so much sense to buy a shoe that fits our foot right at every age, rather than forcing our foot into a shoe.

CHAPTER 12

PODO PROBLEM-SOLVING

PART OF MY GOAL IN WRITING THIS BOOK IS THAT THROUGH educating you as the parent your children will have a different future, hopefully without pain or discomfort.

As a parent it is natural to be concerned if something doesn't look quite right, or your infant is slower than others at reaching milestones or with development. Parents' concerns are often related to what are normal transitions through the milestones. So that will be our focus here: what you're observing, when and what, if anything, to do about it.

CLUB FOOT

Club foot (*talipes equinovarus*) is a congenital (present at birth) condition where one or both feet is turned inwards to give a defined C-shape (IMAGE 12.1).

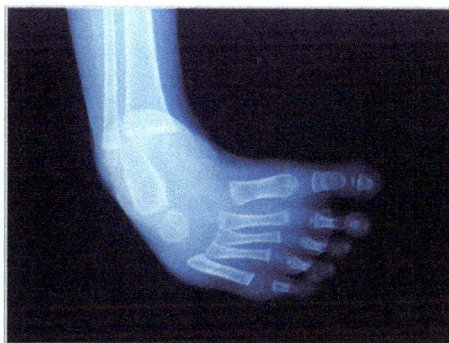

IMAGE 12.1: Club foot (talipes equinovarus).

Cause

Club foot is seen in approximately 1 in every 1,000 births and the cause is unknown. It can be seen in utero, however, it is formally diagnosed after birth and one cause is believed to be shortening of the Achilles tendon. Fetal position and in utero environment (less space/fluid) may also be causal factors. There are variations depending on dominant structures (bones/muscles/tendons) and how they are positioned. Conditions such as spina bifida and cerebral palsy may also present with club foot (neurogenic) and some syndromes can present with club foot (syndromic).

Treatment

Once diagnosed at birth a treatment plan will follow depending on the severity of the club foot presentation. Options will range from soft tissue manipulation and physical therapy, casting and braces, with surgery for the more severe cases.

'I have always found massage to be a vital part of the conventional treatment. A surgeon from USA told a mother who had been in my class that her baby would have needed surgery if she had not been vigilant with her daily feet massage routine.' **CHERRY BOND, NEONATAL EDUCATOR AND CERTIFIED INFANT MASSAGE INSTRUCTOR (IAIM)**

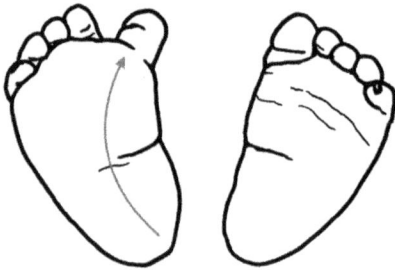

IMAGE 12.2: Metatarsus adductus.

METATARSUS ADDUCTUS

Metatarsus adductus (MA) **(IMAGE 12.2)** is a very mild form of club foot that usually resolves naturally by the age of two. The metatarsal bones are the long bones of the foot, and adduct means to go towards the midline of the body, causing a curved appearance to the foot, high arch and often there is a noticeable gap between the big and second toes.

Cause

Similar to club foot definite causes are unknown, the most likely cause being fetal position in utero. MA is often picked up at birth or shortly after. If not, once the infant is more mobile it may be observed as 'in-toeing' (see page 155).

Developmental dysplasia of the hip (see page 161) is often associated with MA.

Treatment
With MA, there is more chance of this condition resolving naturally if the foot is stimulated through physical therapy such as massage, and once the child is active, spending time barefoot on a wide range of surfaces to encourage their foot to weight bear and build strength. In some cases casts, braces, or special footwear will be used, with surgery for more severe cases.

Activities to help reduce MA
Gentle massage of the leg and foot can help in the early days, stroking the foot into shape (with minimal force). Once the infant is mobile keeping the foot free and experiencing different surfaces will help develop strength and mobility.

PIGEON TOES

The term 'pigeon toed' was originally used in the 1800s to describe a person's foot when the toes pointed in when they walked, also called in-toeing.

In-toeing may develop during infancy (IMAGE 12.3). Assessing which part of the leg and foot is causing it is important. Alignment of the foot bones (metatarsals) may contribute

IMAGE 12.3: In-toeing.

to in-toeing, or rotation of the lower leg (tibia) or upper leg (femur) can also cause in-toeing at the foot.

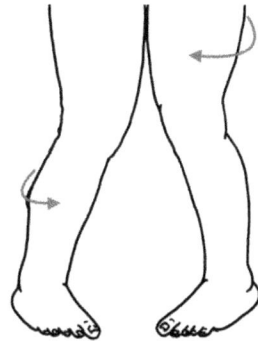

Rotation of leg bones

Internal tibial torsion (ITT) a twisting inwards of the tibia bone of the lower leg (IMAGE 12.3). The knee will look straight and the most visible sign of ITT is in-toeing. This can present in one or both legs and may only become visible upon walking. Rotations of this kind most often naturally resolve by the age of four years.

Femoral anteversion (FA) is where the thigh bone (femur) internally rotates, causing the knees and feet to turn inwards (IMAGE 12.3). FA is usually seen in older children (four to ten years) and like MA and ITT, should naturally resolve. Signs of FA are in-toeing, bowlegs and the child sitting in a 'W' shape.

Cause

Lack of space or positioning in utero is believed to be the main cause of ITT and FA. Sitting in a 'W' shape, a sign of FA, has also been linked to the retained symmetrical tonic neck reflex (see page 39).

Treatment

Physical therapy to strengthen and help with balance is widely used, whereas correcting devices such as orthotics, braces and shoes are ineffective. In severe cases surgery may be an option.

Activities to help reduce ITT/FA

Aside from allowing the infant to develop their own strength as they progress through the milestones, allowing the infant to be barefoot as much as possible will encourage better foot function and improve the relationship between the foot – especially the heel – ankle bone and the lower leg bones, with a flow on effect up the leg. Any barefoot activity and sensory stimulation such as massage may also be beneficial.

Whatever the reason for in-toeing, stimulation and activation of the feet and legs will surely help. Allowing the legs and feet to be free when sleeping could also be of benefit, as could playtime for pre-walkers where they can push their feet flat against the end of their cot or a wall, chair or similar structure.

Seek help at any stage if you are concerned or observe frequent tripping, fatigue or imbalance in walking and physical activity.

BOWLEGS

Bowlegs (*genu varum*) are a normal part of growth and development in the first two years and will generally resolve naturally. You may notice when you are changing your baby's nappies that when you hold both ankles, the legs are not and cannot fully straighten (**IMAGE 12.4**).

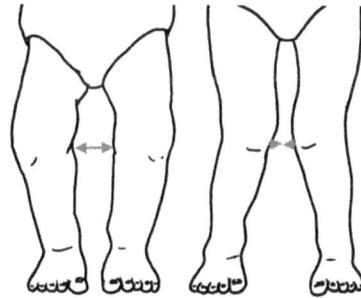

IMAGE 12.4: Bowlegs (left) and knock knees (right).

Cause

Again lack of space in the womb causes the leg bones to rotate slightly.

If the bowlegs persist beyond three years of age, seek advice from your health professional.

KNOCK KNEES

Knock knees (*genu valgum*) appear with knees touching and ankles being further apart, the feet turning outwards. It is again a normal part of a child's growth and development, appearing around two to three years of age. As the foot matures, mobility increases and bones get stronger the legs should straighten at around six to seven years.

Cause

There is no known cause. It is thought that obesity can contribute to knock knees.

Treatment

No treatment is usually necessary for either infant bowlegs or knock knees. Seek advice if knock knees do not resolve, if they appear around six years of age, and if you notice the following:

- asymmetry in their legs
- they complain of pain during activity
- they appear clumsy or are often tired.

Activities to help reduce bowlegs/knock knees

Over time with physical activity, the legs of most children with bowlegs or knock knees will naturally strengthen and straighten. Massaging their feet and legs can be beneficial.

FLAT FEET

Babies are born with juicy fat pads in the midfoot, hiding any presence of the medial longitudinal arch (MLA). We know that the bones that will form the arch in the midfoot are immature at birth, so the absence of arches (*pes planus*) is normal.

Given every opportunity to develop strong healthy feet through the natural movement and the sensory stimulation feet are designed for, arches should develop as the feet mature by your child's tenth birthday.

There may be a structural issue that needs addressing and assessment if, when your child starts school, you have concerns about their arches, or if you notice the following:

- their left and right feet look different
- they complain of pain during activity
- they are clumsy.

Observation and monitoring may be the first steps until the foot matures, as in many cases flat feet will spontaneously resolve.

TOE-WALKING

It is fairly common for the novice walker to cruise and totter around up on the balls of their feet (IMAGE 12.5). As they gain confidence, toe-walking may linger and it will appear like they have a bouncy walk where their heel doesn't land at all.

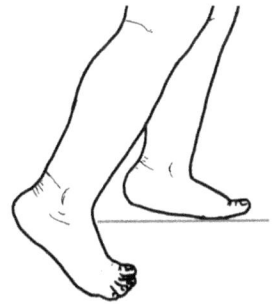

Infants will usually outgrow this pattern of walking by the age of five years.

IMAGE 12.5: Toe-walking.

Cause
The cause is really unknown (idiopathic) and may vary from infant to infant. Possible reasons for toe-walking are:

- Growth spurts. Bones grow longer stretching the muscles, so to relieve this the infant rises up to reduce tension.
- Sensitivity. Infants that were premature are sometimes hypersensitive in the heel due to the many heel pricks they experienced in hospital; other infants may lack tolerance for different reasons.
- Sensory-seeking. Up on their toes, infants increase their proprioceptive input.
- Unintegrated primitive reflexes such as the tonic labyrinthine reflex (TLR) or Babinski (see pages 42 and 36).

- Inactivity.
- Toe-walking may also be an early sign of cerebral palsy and muscular dystrophy, and has been linked to autism.

Treatment

Persistent or asymmetrical (one-sided) toe-walking beyond three years should be checked out for peace of mind as there may be an underlying neurological or developmental reason. Early intervention offered may include physio or physical therapy and special footwear. Without early intervention, botox injections, casts or surgery may be the only solutions as the child gets older. Often it is the physical presentation/ condition/symptom that is treated, but with the knowledge of primitive and postural reflexes shared in this book, you may benefit from checking these first.

Any change to an infant's posture and movement may lead to postural adaptations and imbalances, which may then cause:

- muscle weakness and fatigue
- clumsiness
- pain
- vision problems
- social stigma.

Activities to help prevent and reduce toe-walking

Prevention is better than cure, so rather than waiting to see if your infant will toe-walk here's some ideas (these activities can also be used after toe-walking has started):

- Gentle stimulation to the soles of their feet with massage and touch, allowing their feet to have a variety of input.
- Encouraging activity through play can help 'ground' your infant's feet, e.g., squatting and climbing both encourage the heel to

drop. Balance activities like standing on one leg, walking on their heels plus getting outside on different surfaces and walking uphill may be of benefit. And don't forget those shoes with squeaky heels.

DEVELOPMENTAL DYSPLASIA OF THE HIP (DDH)

Dysplasia refers to abnormal growth or development, in this case of the hip joint where the femur joins the pelvis. It is routinely checked for at birth by assessing hip movement and comparing left and right sides for anomalies such as leg length and skin creases.

Cause
Positioning and lack of space in the womb can be a contributing factor, and in some cases it may be genetic.

Treatment
If DDH is suspected at birth, this will be followed up during routine medical checks. In most babies, DDH resolves within the first two to three months as they grow and their bones harden. For others, early treatment involves a soft brace to support correct alignment and growth.

Activities to help DDH
- Allowing your baby plenty of floor time with their legs and feet free to move and kick.
- Not swaddling them too tightly especially around the hips and legs.
- Using only socks to avoid any extra weight on their legs.
- Gently massaging and moving the baby's legs.

CONDITIONS OF THE TOES

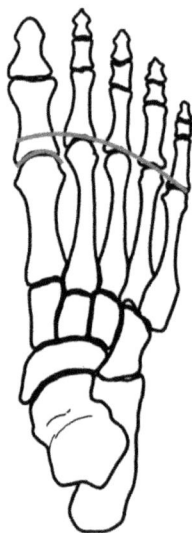

IMAGE 12.6: Morton's toe.

SYNDACTYLY, also known as zygodactyly, presents as webbed toes at birth, often between the second and third toes. Unless it causes pain or affects function, no treatment is necessary.

POLYDACTYLY is where there is an extra toe. If it causes a problem it may be removed after an infant's first birthday.

MORTON'S TOE (named after surgeon Dudley Morton) is when the first metatarsal bone is shorter than the second metatarsal (**IMAGE 12.6**). As a result, the second toe may appear longer than the big toe but it's at the joint where the metatarsal (long bone) meets the small toe bones that needs checking. This congenital anomaly may impact walking, shifting the propulsion force to the second and third toes. This is a structural condition that most people live with, requiring no treatment. I would strongly encourage shoes with a wide toe box so as not to put extra pressure on the big toe.

HAMMER TOE presents as an abnormal bend in the middle joints most commonly of the second, third and fourth toes. Wearing shoes with a flat and wide toe box is recommended.

MALLET TOE affects the most distal, end joint, again of the second, third and fourth toes. My son Nick had mallet toes in both feet. It didn't seem to affect him, but it didn't look normal. Looking back, I wonder if he developed them because I didn't change his shoes as his feet grew, or if there was something else going on in his posture that had him gripping the ground? Perhaps a retained plantar reflex? He was eleven years old when I finally took some time and treated him. But where to start, what to do? My friend who introduced me to fascia suggested an imbalance between his front and back causing him to grip with his toes. He also had the start of a forward head posture (and this was pre-electronic devices!). I worked to bring balance to his overall system. The results were great (given I was inexperienced at this point!). Not only was there a change in his toes but his overall posture changed. I would love to wind the clock back. There's so much more I would have explored with him. The best thing I can do now is help you and other parents **(IMAGES 12.7 & 12.8)**.

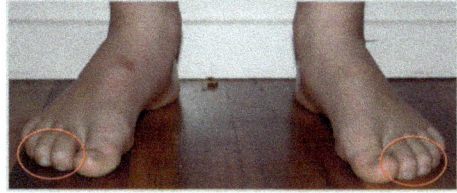

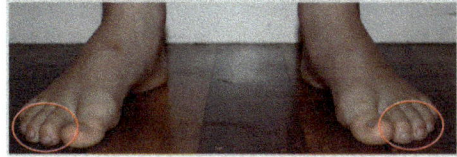

IMAGES 12.7 & 12.8: Nick's toes before and after fascial treatment. Before, the second, third and fourth toes are curled under and you can hardly see the toenails. The toenails start emerging after a series of treatments. (Photo: B Landels)

Picking up on toe deformities such as mallet and hammer toe early is important and could avoid invasive corrective procedures later in life.

And we need to think beyond just the toes, knowing that our fascial system connects everything. If there is a problem in the foot we must check the rest of the body, and vice versa. Some postural issues, tension and pain originate from poor biomechanics in the feet.

Foot care and care of our foundation of support is crucial during infancy and childhood. And don't forget about the nails.

FOOTCARE

Keeping nails trimmed, washing in-between and under the toes, and removing lint from socks is the hands-on care tiny feet need. The other care is hands-off! Or should that be shoes-off! And you should NEVER see marks from socks or shoes on little feet; if you do, REMOVE them. They are not the right shape or size.

ANKLE SPRAINS

Ankle sprains don't really fit in this list, but I thought I would throw it in because statistics report that it is one of the most common injuries of the lower leg in adults. And, as my book is about prevention, I want to plant an idea with you. If your child grows up spending more time barefoot or in minimalistic footwear, developing a strong and adaptable foundation, with good proprioceptive and vestibular feedback loops, sensory awareness and perception, would that reduce their chances of ankle sprain later on?

The most common ankle sprain occurs when you roll outwards on the ankle, straining the ligaments on the outside of the ankle beyond their natural limits. If the tissues were adaptable, and had experienced a full range of motion growing up, then the outcome may be different.

When we limit movement, weakness and reduced adaptability result, so time spent barefoot doing a wide range of activities on different surfaces and terrain, i.e., playing, may prevent injuries such as sprains.

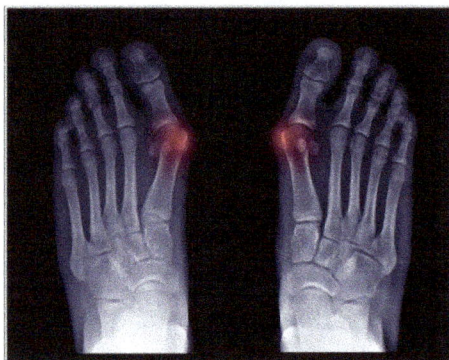

IMAGE 12.9: X-ray image of adult feet showing the angling and rotation of the first metatarsal bones. The toe bones only have one option and that is to turn outwards. The red highlights where the 'bunion' appears but not necessarily where the problem lies.

BUNION BONUS

I know for sure that infants do not have bunions, but there have been reports that 2% of children aged nine to ten start to develop them.[46] So again I am going to play the prevention card here.

A bunion (*hallux valgus*) is an often-painful swollen 'bump' just below the big toe at the first metatarsophalangeal joint (MTPJ) **(IMAGE 12.9).**

Cause

The bump is caused by the big toe angling outwards, towards the second toe and the inner aspect of the joint opening too much. The question is – what causes the big toe to angle out? Often the issue is not with the toe joint itself. The mis-alignment may be a result of poor biomechanics or posture changing the force into the joint, causing the joint to become unstable. The answer may also lie in the plasticity of the tissues, and years of wearing ill-fitting shoes that have restricted the foot and directed the force during movement into the joint, causing the toe to turn outwards. Or it may be a combination of both!

You may have also thought that if your parent had/has them, they must be hereditary. Maybe there's some truth there; it may be similar body type or genetics. However, think back to Katja's story (page 103) and how her little boy copied Katja and his dad. Can you see how you may have potentially copied your parents' movement patterns as well? Imitation may lay down the lines of stress and tension that may present in something like a bunion.

Treatment

People usually do not seek treatment for bunions until they are in pain, and by then it may be too late. Standard/conventional treatment involves addressing the MTPJ in isolation with toe spreaders, splints, pads and – failing all else – surgery. I have seen the results of too many surgeries to sit idle and not share what I know – hence this book about your baby and this part of the chapter for you. Surgery should only be considered as a last resort once all other options are exhausted.

Treatment should start with an assessment of biomechanics, how your whole body moves in relation to your feet. Look beyond the pain and bump to work out what is or isn't happening. Footwear, as we know, impacts our posture and movement so this too needs addressing.

See resources page 187 for information on recommended health professionals and services.

Activities to help prevent or reduce bunions

Every foot is different and so it is hard to provide a comprehensive list of activities ... awareness and prevention are key. The health of your feet is important for your overall health and wellbeing. Use the following QR code to visit the resources page of my website, and check out my 5 Minute Foot Blasts and other movement cues to re-awaken your feet and body.

Here's a chart to summarise conditions that should resolve naturally and how you can help:

Condition	Age observed	Check if not resolved by	Will benefit from barefoot physical activity	Massage & stimulation of foot may help
Metatarsus adductus	0–2 yrs	2 yrs	Yes	Yes
Internal tibial torsion	0–4 yrs	4 yrs	Yes	Yes
Femoral anteversion	4–10 yrs	10 yrs	Yes	Yes
Bowlegs	0–2 yrs	2 yrs	Yes	Yes
Knock knees	2–7 yrs	7 yrs, or if appears around 6 yrs	Yes	Yes
Flat feet	0–10 yrs	10 yrs	Yes	Yes
Toe-walking	Onset of walking–5 yrs	3 yrs	Yes	Yes

PAEDIATRIC FOOT ASSESSMENT

The information in this chapter should not be used as a diagnostic tool, and you should check with your registered health professional if you have any concerns.

If you do seek a professional opinion regarding your child's feet, the assessment may include asking questions relating to the following:

- major milestones – so keep a note of these
- falling/tripping history, and a comparison to siblings
- reported pain in legs or feet
- fatiguing, tiring easily in the foot and lower leg, asking to be carried
- ability to run, jump, hop, etc. (age dependent)
- general health and any other conditions present
- family foot history.

A physical assessment will look for asymmetries in structure and function. These may include the following:

- examination of both feet, palpation of tissues, checking reflexes
- range of motion (passive/active) of joints
- observation standing – all three planes
- video/pressure plate analysis of walking (gait) – both barefoot and with footwear on, again in all three views/planes
- note the angle of tendons, e.g., Achilles
- balance – ability to stand on one leg
- checking footwear.

SHOE INSERTS

Orthopaedic insoles should be a last resort, in my opinion, with young developing bodies. Like a shoe they can weaken the muscles of the foot by stopping any functional movement. They may be necessary to reduce pain whilst further assessment is carried out to find the underlying cause of the issue present, e.g., flat feet or heel pain.

I would strongly encourage parents to seek a second opinion, even a third, if insoles are suggested as the only solution.

If a podiatrist or healthcare professional recommends insoles for your child, ask the following questions:

- What are the inserts designed to do?
- What is not happening in my child's body that is causing the problem?
- How long will they have to wear them?

Remember everything is connected, so a problem in the foot may be from somewhere else that is not moving or moving too much.

The health, growth and development of your child is in your hands.

We have explored your child's physical growth through reflexes, milestones and movement – setting the foundation for all other aspects of what makes them whole. By understanding more about their journey and their body, and the importance of their feet and the floor, you can provide them with the stimulation and opportunities they need and set them up for success.

But wait! There is a little more I'd like to share, so join me as we explore the body a little more through touch ...

BONUS

CHAPTER 13

TOUCH

UNTIL NOW WE'VE BEEN LOOKING AT TOUCH FROM AN EXTERO-
ceptive view. Your baby reached out with feet and hands to explore, interpret and identify their external environments while in the womb and this continues after birth. Touch helps hardwire their neurological map, develop proprioception and awareness of themselves in gravity.

Unlike the glabrous skin on their palms and soles, the rest of your baby's body is covered in soft hairs. In your womb, as they swim around in amniotic fluid, constantly stimulated, their wee hairy body is gently massaged by the watery environment. They will even respond to your touch through your belly more than your voice.

During the birthing process each contraction massages your baby, then a vaginal delivery helps expel fluid from their lungs by this squeezing massage (which is why sometimes with C-section first breaths can be a challenge). Once delivered, hopefully the next touch and squeeze is being held in loving arms. It's pretty scary going from a watery environment to a breezy one; from a cosy hotel with great 'womb' service (couldn't resist slipping that in) to vast open spaces and bright lights; and from being cut from the endless supply of nutrients to having to work for every meal! Skin-to-skin after birth helps reassure your baby and is the beginning of a lifelong communication where exteroception meets interoception (feelings from within). The smells, sights and sounds come flooding in from your baby's new external world, along with your smell and breath, as well as familiar voices. It is an inherently mutual multi-sensory experience, one that conveys your baby belongs.

Touch conveys to your baby that they have a place in this world **(IMAGE 13.1).**

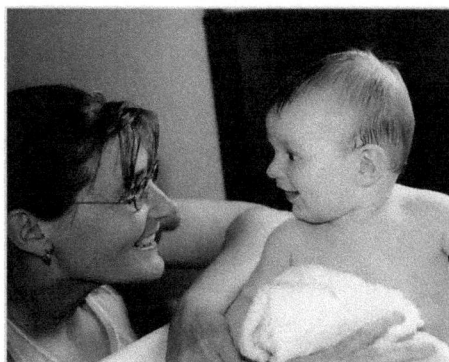

IMAGE 13.1: Ben and I – no words needed. (Photo: L Edgell)

'Touch is a basic need from birth to death.' PEGGY DAWSON

INFANT MASSAGE

Infant massage and gentle movement may help the soft tissues associated with some of the conditions mentioned in the previous chapter. Understanding the nature of our tissue development, connections and layers, we can use touch to possibly bring change and awareness.

You may have heard stories of children in orphanages in the 1980s who were neglected, receiving no affection or touch. Both physical and mental development was severely delayed. One study showed the brains of children who grew up in orphanages in Romania were physically smaller than in healthy children.[47] Tiffany Field, director of the Touch Research Institute, University of Miami School of Medicine, who has been studying touch since the 1990s, calls touch 'the mother of all senses'. In Maslow's hierarchy of needs,[48] touch stands alongside other basic requirements; remove touch and survival becomes a challenge.

Times have definitely changed since the 1980s and are still changing, and as technology advances so does the ability to understand the human body and mind. And yet massage has been around for thousands of years with records from China, India and Egypt dating back to 2700 BCE. Infant massage records are a little sketchy, but it is known that Asian and Pacific Island cultures have a longstanding history of using massage from birth.

As part of my massage training in New Zealand we probably spent the same amount of time studying the history of massage as we did learning about how to massage infants. I didn't have children at that stage so whilst it was interesting, I never used the skills. When I had my son Nick in 2000, I dug up the brief notes and began to give him small massages. I really enjoyed massaging him and I think he enjoyed receiving. I was the massage therapist for the NZ Silver Ferns netball team when Nick was born and continued to travel for a year or so after his birth. The time apart was hard, initially because I kept expressing milk whilst I was away so that I could continue breastfeeding on my return and I missed Nick incredibly. Massage and breastfeeding helped maintain our strong bond during time apart.

During Nick's first years, I opened a new clinic alongside my midwife and expanded into pre and postnatal massage, running workshops for parents, teaching them how to massage each other and sharing massage options for during labour. Parents then started asking me to teach them how to massage their babies, so I went and got myself trained! In 2002, I trained to be an instructor with the International Association of Infant Massage (IAIM), a comprehensive training that taught me a lot more than infant massage. I also added reflexology to my tool kit as a way to work with systems of the body through the feet. Ben was born the next year and having had more experience working with other parents, he could not escape my hands (IMAGE 13.2).

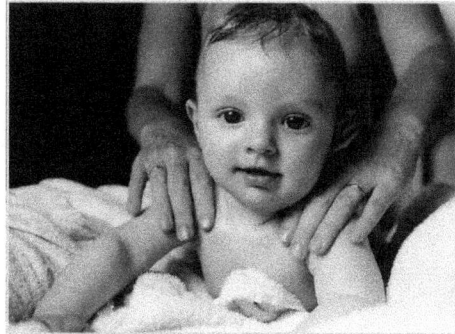

IMAGE 13.2: Ben enjoying a massage after his bath. (Photo: L Edgell)

IAIM was founded in 1986 by Vimala McClure a few years after she spent time in India where she observed and learnt traditional infant massage. Massage was part of all mothers' daily routine there. During my IAIM training, I came across Frederic Leboyer's book *Loving Hands: The Traditional Art of Baby Massage*. He was a French obstetrician and advocate for gentle birthing techniques who also spent time in India. When I saw Leboyer's photos of Indian women sitting on the bare ground, massaging their infant on their outstretched legs, I thought then (and still do today), *what wealth they have compared to us in the Western world.* Although surrounded by such poverty, their culture provides such wealth with the basic needs of loving, nurturing touch being met from the very beginning of life.

IAIM is now internationally renowned with Certified Infant Massage Instructors (CIMI) in over fifty countries around the world. Their mission statement: *The purpose of IAIM is to promote nurturing touch and communication through training, education and research so that parents, caregivers and their children are loved, valued, and respected throughout the world community.*

BENEFITS OF TOUCH

Research and anecdotal evidence provide a solid base from which to understand the wide-ranging possible benefits of massaging your infant from birth and throughout their childhood.

Let's unpack some of the benefits by dipping back into the brain and body for a moment to understand what happens when you touch and massage your infant.

At birth, your baby's nervous system is immature, not fully developed. Stimulation through massage will hasten the process of myelination, the growth of the sheath that covers nerves, speeding up the transmission of the all-important messages from as far afield as your baby's soles to their brain. This forms an important body–brain connection for spatial awareness, coordination and proprioception.

Housed in the fascia below your baby's skin covered with soft hairs, your baby has special C-tactile low-threshold mechanoreceptors (C-LTMRs). These nerves are un-myelinated, so messages from them travel more slowly to the brain. They also take a more circuitous route than other nerves I've talked about, going via the thalamus (the brain's 'gatekeeper' of sensory information), to the hypothalamus (part of the brain which produces particular hormones), to the insular cortex (part of the brain involved in inner perception). The response to being touched by you, or another person, is quite different to when they reached out with their hands and feet.

These C-LTMRs respond to touch that is light, slow and warm. It's a bit of a Goldilocks moment – not too deep, nor too light, just enough to move their skin. And we are talking a stroke of 3–5 cm per second. Stroke your index finger from knuckle to tip and count 'one and'. The ideal temperature is warm, like how our skin feels, around 32 degrees.

Underneath their skin the C-LTMRs come alive, sending messages to various parts of the brain and the floodgates open. Dopamine, oxytocin, serotonin and endorphins (think a good DOSE) are released into the brain and bloodstream. These hormones provide many benefits, from helping with sleep and digestion to bonding. Let's take a closer look at what a good DOSE will do.[49]

Dopamine is a 'feel-good' chemical, released from three different parts of our brain, including the hypothalamus. Once your infant has learnt the signals for when a massage is about to start, even anticipation can boost their levels of dopamine. This chemical is released into different parts of the brain such as the hippocampus (which stores memory), creating massage memories and the desire for more.

Oxytocin is widely known as the 'love' hormone. Secreted by the pituitary gland, it's also released during orgasm, labour and lactation (breastfeeding), and it is an important factor in bonding development. It also lowers blood pressure and stress levels.

Serotonin is another 'feel-good' chemical that is produced by the brain stem and by the digestive tract, levels increasing with loving touch. It helps stabilise mood and promotes feelings of happiness. It also helps with sleep and digestion. With most of the serotonin in your stomach and intestines, it's possibly where our 'gut feeling' comes from.

Endorphins are produced naturally by eating dark chocolate. (Nothing to do with massage, I know. I love dark chocolate. It's good for your health!) Seriously though, endorphins, released during massage into the bloodstream by the pituitary gland, are natural painkillers and boost pleasure and relaxation. They help reinforce attachment and give a natural 'high'.

Another hormone worth mentioning here is cortisol which is the stress hormone produced in the hypothalamus and the pituitary and adrenal glands. It has been found that massage helps lower levels in the blood. Stress drives levels up and high levels of cortisol have been found to have negative effects on immune function. At birth your baby's immune system is immature but adaptive. Massage may reduce cortisol levels. It has also been found that massage increases the number of white blood cells (lymphocytes) that help the body fight infection and disease. So, massage is a winner for both stress and immunity.

To further understand touch, we need to expand our knowledge of the nervous system a little more. Many of the topics we have looked at in this book so far have involved the central nervous system, the development of feedback loops relating to movement and sensory input as a baby grows.

There is another branch of the nervous system called the 'autonomic nervous system' (ANS). The ANS regulates our internal organs and involuntary processes, such as digestion and breathing. It is divided into two opposite systems (parasympathetic and sympathetic) which bring balance to our body. The sympathetic system controls 'fight or flight', our response to stress and danger, whilst the parasympathetic nervous system (PNS) controls our relaxation response which is important for rest, digestion and healing.[50]

Loving, positive touch not only starts a cascade of hormones, it sends messages to the brain to activate the PNS. Researchers at the Touch Research Institute, University of Miami School of Medicine, found that the key player in regulating the PNS was the vagus nerve, which is the longest and most widespread cranial nerve in the body.[51] These researchers found that vagal activity increased following infant massage, which in turn calmed the baby and stimulated digestion through the release of food-absorption hormones such as gastrin and insulin. This is one reason why massage, received several times a day, promotes weight gain in pre-term infants.

Infant massage may also help reduce the effects of colic and reflux. Think about this common scenario faced by at least a quarter of all parents: the fussy, hard to settle, gassy, crying baby that may have been labelled as 'colicky', or suffering from infantile colic.

Colic is the term used when a healthy baby cries inconsolably for long periods, presumably from pain in their abdomen originating in the colon. But the cause of this distress is unknown, and the diagnosis is made on behaviours, such as extreme crying. Other causes have been proposed, such as allergies or maternal diet if breastfeeding, or hyper-sensitivity to changes either in their body or their environment. Not only is your baby born with an immature nervous system, their digestive system is not fully mature at birth either. They have to switch supply from the placenta to an external source of nutrients (breast or bottle) and start digesting, absorbing and producing enzymes, all in a matter of moments. This immaturity has also been used to explain the occurrence of 'colic' (poor digestion and wind) in babies in the first three to four months. Even over-anxious parents have been attributed to colic. As you can imagine or may have experienced, the crying associated with colic does nothing for one's stress levels or emotions, let alone your relationship with your baby, partner and other family members.

If we look at the behaviour – crying – the reason a baby will cry is because of physical or emotional needs. They may be hungry, have a dirty nappy, be too hot or cold, or be in pain. They may be frightened, lonely, over- or under-stimulated, even bored. Crying is their way of getting your attention and having their needs met.

In addition to crying, a baby with colic may appear stiff and tense, with a distended (swollen) belly, and may draw their knees up to their belly or arch their back. These may be signs that they are uncomfortable.

Suggested treatments range from massage, rocking and warm baths to anti-colic drops, herbal remedies and changing the mother's diet. And because each wee baby is different, what works for one may not work for another – basically there's no known cure. Having experienced the despair, the helplessness, as Nick cried, and having tried every remedy I could think of and that was suggested to me, I feel it's right to reach out to you and share what I know now. The first thing you need to know: it's not your fault. But why wait for it to develop – can we help prevent your baby from these crying episodes?

Rhythmic movement (such as rocking and being carried) and vibrations (such as going for a ride in the car or resting on the parent's chest) can calm a baby, even put them to sleep. A warm bath and 'white noise' are also calming. These all provide familiar sensations from being inside the womb and yet with a 'colicky' baby often none of these work, or work whilst happening but the moment you put them down or stop the movement, they start screaming again. These are great options, to a point, but wouldn't it be better to reduce these occurrences? Think of it like filling up your car with fuel so that you don't run out. Let me explain – regular massage and positive, nurturing touch fills your baby so they don't 'run out' and scream for more ... and there is little point waiting until they run out to do something.

I have already mentioned the effect touch can have on certain hormones. Massage helps release endorphins, the natural painkillers that also induce relaxation. So massage would help if the colic was causing pain. Oxytocin and cortisol lower stress levels; if your baby is crying, both your and their stress levels would be heightened. Serotonin levels are increased through massage, which aids digestion and has a positive effect on mood, as does dopamine. If you want to use massage to calm an upset baby, they need to have experienced it when you are both calm, when you are both in the mood, when they are not screaming and you are not tearing your hair out and reaching for the earmuffs.

Massage helps calm the nerves, literally; add in slow breathing, humming and a soothing voice and you'll have the attention of the vagus nerve, and their PNS will develop a stronger relaxation response. We need to teach our baby how to relax, through touch, sounds and our facial expressions. The vagus nerve can also be activated with gentle movement (see page 49), time outside in nature and gargling – all part of the great family diet.

What about reflux? Reflux is when a baby spills or is sick during or after feeding. Again, we could attribute it to an immature digestive tract where the structures between the oesophagus (food pipe) and stomach are not fully developed, or if you are in too much of a hurry to wind baby, whatever is above a 'wind bubble' and has not made it to the stomach will come back up. Here you need to think of the baby's oesophagus like a spirit level, and slowly tilt baby so that the bubble slides up and out before any milk does. And of course then there's the vagus nerve – drum roll please. The vagus nerve innervates the muscles responsible for swallowing, so it may be possible that if massage stimulates the vagus nerve, the muscles can do their job better.

Like the importance of feet as our foundation, positive nurturing touch can set the scene for a happy, healthy sense of well-being. And like walking barefoot on uneven terrain and rough ground increases your infant's tolerance for their external world, daily massage will increase their threshold for stimulation and foster their internal world.

I also believe that giving your infant a regular massage will help you become more aware of their body. You may notice tension or asymmetries earlier, even before walking. Then once they are walking, you will have a sharper eye and, with knowledge from this book, a greater understanding of how the body develops and moves.

Benefits of infant massage
- Improves body awareness and coordination.
- Increases threshold for stimulation.

- Produces a good DOSE of hormones to help with:
  - bonding
  - mood
  - relaxation
  - sleep and digestion
  - reducing pain
  - improving immunity
  - reducing colic and reflux
  - weight gain.

Benefits for you, the parents
- Builds confidence and self esteem through learning new skills.
- Enhances bonding with your baby.
- May even alleviate symptoms of post-natal depression.

Massage is for all the family to be involved in.

Another great benefit is your infant will learn through receiving and one day may massage you in return. I was collecting Ben from childcare one day and he was outside with the other children and his teacher. She was sitting on the mini trampoline, and the children were taking turns to push on her shoulders to make her bounce, until it was Ben's turn. I saw him say something and then give her a shoulder massage. My heart melted as I realised Ben's experience of being massaged had had such an impact on him that he wanted to share it.

You cannot touch without being touched.

INTRODUCTION TO INFANT MASSAGE

Imagine your infant in a warm room, lying on a blanket with no distractions, no noise apart from breathing or maybe some gentle music playing in the background. You make eye contact with your baby and show them your warm caring hands. You swish some oil between your hands to warm it and ask your baby if they would like a massage. These are all cues for your baby to learn it's massage time.

Of course, your infant can't reply verbally when they are very young but they have ways to let you know they're ready such as bright eye contact and smiling face or an enthusiastic kick and open arms trying to embrace what is about to happen.

Or perhaps it's not the right time for them; they will let you know by turning their eyes away, rolling away, turning their back to you, and of course, crying. Pick them up, cuddle them or tend to their other needs. This is a very important aspect of touch to teach your infant. If someone wants to touch them, they are the ones to give permission; they have a choice. Try again later.

You can establish a routine of when you will massage your infant, or integrate it with bath time. You can also grab moments where you may just massage their hands, feet or face. Infant massage is a portable skill that can last a few minutes or longer. The first holiday we went on after Nick was born, we forgot the key to the house, so while waiting for friends to bring the key, I stripped Nick off and sat in the sun giving him a massage (IMAGE 13.3).

It is best to massage with an unscented plant oil such as sunflower or coconut. Oils such as

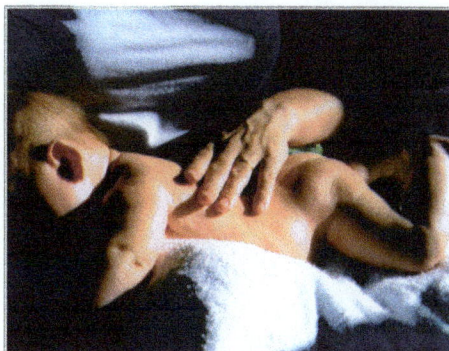

IMAGE 13.3: Nick bares all for a massage in the sun. (Photo: K Bevin)

grapeseed can be good if there are allergies. Organic and cold-pressed (no heat or chemicals used in production) is recommended. Whilst these can be expensive, you use very little when massaging so they do last.

One-to-one focused exchange begins, and interoception increases as your infant feels your touch, hands gently touching their skin, sensing temperature, texture and tension as your hands move, starting at the feet and legs.

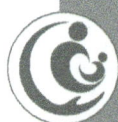

LEG MASSAGE

Use this QR code to visit the resources page of my website, where you can view a video of the following routine.

The legs and feet are a perfect part of your infant's body to introduce massage as you handle and expose them throughout the day when you change their nappy. And as we have seen, the legs and feet are an important part of the body.

So get yourself and your infant comfortable by laying them on their back, asking if they would like a massage, and swishing the oil in your hands. Now let's begin.

Rest your warm hands on their legs. This tells them where you are going to massage, like saying hello.

Your speed will be slow and pressure 'just right'. Repeat each stroke several times on each side. At first your infant may only tolerate a short massage, so use fewer strokes.

Top to bottom
Take one leg and stroke downwards from their hip to their foot with one hand. You will find your hand cups around

their leg in a C-shape. Repeat with your other hand and repeat the strokes several times. Repeat on the other leg.

Bottom of foot

Holding one foot, use your thumbs to sweep one after the other from heel to toes on the sole of their foot. You can also press your thumbs gently into their sole. You may notice the plantar or Babinski reflexes in action as you do this. Repeat on the other foot.

Toes

Gently roll each toe between your thumb and first finger. This is a great time to introduce any rhymes or songs such as 'This little piggy went to market'.

This is an ideal time to check the small creases and between the toes for any sock fluff!

Top of foot

Cradle their heel in your fingers whilst you stroke with alternating thumbs from toes to ankle on the top of their foot. Repeat on the other foot.

Ankle

Still holding their foot in your fingertips, use both thumbs in a circular action all around their tiny ankle. Repeat on other ankle.

Bottom to top

Sweep your C-shaped hands from their foot to hip one after the other, repeating on the other leg after a few strokes.

Roll

Holding one leg between both palms, roll their leg left and right so their leg rotates a little each way with the movement. You can start at the hip and move down to the foot with this movement. Repeat on the other leg.

Relax

Holding both feet in your hands, gently lift and lower their legs. Tell them gently to relax as you lower their legs and see if they can let their legs be heavy. Praise them when they do.

Complete the massage by slowly wrapping or dressing them, and relax with them for a moment before you do anything else.

To learn a full massage visit IAIM (see link on resources page 187) to find an instructor near you, or reach out into your community; there are bound to be classes being run. If not, contact me!

REFLEXOLOGY

The foot is an amazing structure, as we have seen as we walked through this book together. I cannot avoid mentioning the ancient art of reflexology where the whole body is reflected in the feet (also hands and ears).

Reflexology has similar origins to that of massage dating back to the ancient cultures of Egypt, China, India, Japan and Europe. Modern reflexology dates back to the 1900s with the well-known work of Dr William Fitzgerald (1872–1942). Eunice Ingham (1879–1974) was another pioneer of the practice, and whose work the Ingham method of reflexology is based on.

As a complementary health option, reflexology has been used widely to treat many health problems as it is safe and appears to be effective, despite the lack of evidence-based studies to back it up.

There are many reported benefits of how reflexology can improve well-being, but what about your infant? I went on the hunt for some current literature and found a systematic review published in 2020 reporting on the effects of reflexology on child health.[52] The authors' review of all the literature resulted in their concluding that reflexology can reduce acute pain and infantile colic symptoms. I believe this links back to the effect of touch on the nervous system, how touch can help maturation, and how the release of endorphins are our natural painkillers and relaxants (IMAGE 13.4).

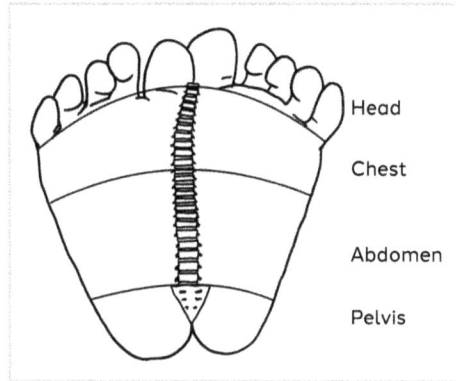

IMAGE 13.4: How the body is divided up in the foot according to reflexology.

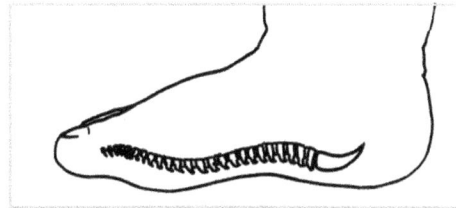

IMAGE 13.5: Is the spine reflected in the foot shape? Does healthy foot movement create a healthy spine?

I do wonder now though if there is in fact a structural connection to reflexology. Walking barefoot is surely a natural stimulant to the reflex points.

Now we know that for a healthy foot we need the arch to pronate (lengthen and open) and supinate (close and twist). These movements create a 3D chain reaction all the way up the body, so if your foot is not moving well neither is your spine, your organs, or your head. If you see where the spinal column is depicted on the foot (IMAGE 13.5), one question comes to mind: is there a connection?'

Maybe that's my next book!

RESOURCES

Knowing where to start to look for information can be daunting. This list gives you details of international organisations relating to topics in *Finding Their Feet*, and where you can find links to practitioners and further help.

Infant massage
Not only can you find a class on how to learn to give massage, it may open up doors for you to become a certified instructor and teach other parents.

https://iaim.net

Primitive reflexes
While there are a number of good online resources about primitive reflexes, if you are concerned about your infant it is best to find a reputable practitioner for a complete assessment. Here are a few places to start:

https://www.rhythmicmovement.org/consultants

https://www.drrobertmelillo.com/referrals

https://www.smartlearning.co.nz/practitioners

Infant treatment
When looking for any health professional to help with your baby, ensure they are qualified and experienced in paediatrics, i.e., working

with babies and children. Whether they are a chiropractor, osteopath or podiatrist/chiropodist, ask about their treatment, approach and success stories to ensure they are who you and your child need.

Adult foot problems

As many adult foot problems stem from something somewhere else in the body then I would suggest the following options:

Structural Integration (SI): These practitioners work the whole body, looking at your alignment. Working with your fascia, getting to the layers that may be stuck rather than just massaging muscles, this work can bring more ease and freedom to your whole body. Look for qualified Anatomy Trains (ATSI) or Kinesis Myofascial Integration (KMI) practitioners or trained Rolfers. These are all different brands of SI. Some SI practitioners also work with children.

https://iasi.memberclicks.net/find-a-practitioner

https://www.anatomytrains.com/practitioners

https://rolfing.org/find-rolfer

https://mms.rolf.org/members/directory/search_rolf_FAR.php

Anatomy in Motion: Based on the work of Gary Ward, author of *What the Foot*, practitioners work with your posture and how you move. Looking at relationships between your body and feet.
https://findingcentre.co.uk/find-help

 To explore a list of resources and books for additional reading and information, please use this QR code to visit my website, www.bernielandels.com/resources.

AN OVERVIEW OF PRIMITIVE REFLEXES

Reflex	Pregnancy – Trimesters			Birth	First year – months											
	1st	2nd	3rd		1	2	3	4	5	6	7	8	9	10	11	12
1 Moro	Wk 10															
2 Plantar	Wk 10															
3 Babinski	Wk 10															
4 Stepping			Wk 37													
5 ATNR		Wk 20														
6 Bauer			Wk 28													
7 Spinal Galant		Wk 20														
8 TLR	Wk 12															
9 Landau																
10 STNR																

Emerge | Develop | Integrate

Primitive reflexes (1–8) emerge during pregnancy, develop into movement patterns for training of the body and brain, before integrating and transforming into postural reflexes and voluntary movements. The Landau and STNR are actually transitional reflexes that help the infant move from one stage to another. The TLR and Landau remain in a weakened form for up to three years. The above timeframes are a guide only, variations will occur with each baby depending on their in utero/birth experience and opportunity for movement in their first year.

ENDNOTES

1   World Health Organization, *Monitoring Children's Development in the Primary Care Services: Moving from a Focus on Child Deficits to Family-Centred Participatory Support. Report of a Virtual Technical Meeting, 9–10 June 2020* (Geneva: World Health Organization, 2020), vii, https://www.who.int/publications/i/item/9789240012479.

2   Robert Schleip, 'Fascia as an Organ of Communication,' in *Fascia: The Tensional Network of the Human Body*, eds. Robert Schleip, Peter Huijing, Leon Chaitow, and Thomas W. Findley (London: Churchill Livingstone, 2012), 77–79.

3   Stewart C. Morrison et al., 'Time to Revise Our Dialogue: How *Flat* is the Paediatric *Flat*foot?" *Journal of Foot and Ankle Research* 10, article no. 50 (2017), https://doi.org/10.1186/s13047-017-0233-2.

4   John D. Nguyen and Hieu Duong, *Neurosurgery, Sensory Homunculus* (Treasure Island, FL: StatPearls Publishing, 2021), https://www.ncbi.nlm.nih.gov/books/NBK549841.

5   Sandra Ackerman, 'The Development and Shaping of the Brain,' in *Discovering the Brain* (Washington: National Academies Press, 1992), 86–103, https://www.ncbi.nlm.nih.gov/books/NBK234146.

6   Robert Schleip, 'Innervation of Fascia,' in *Fascia, Function, and Medical Applications*, eds. David Lesondak and Angeli Maun Akey (Boca Raton: CRC Press, 2021), 61.

7   Kimberley Whitehead, Judith Meek, and Lorenzo Fabrizi, 'Developmental Trajectory of Movement-Related Cortical Oscillations During Active Sleep in a Cross-Sectional Cohort of Pre-Term and Full-Term Human Infants,' *Scientific Reports* 8, article no. 17516 (2018), https://doi.org/10.1038/s41598-018-35850-1.

8   Sally Goddard Blyth, *The Well Balanced Child: Movement and Early Learning* (Gloucestershire: Hawthorn Press, 2005), 24.

9 'Millennium Cohort Study,' Centre for Longitudinal Studies, University College London, last modified 26 October, 2021, https://cls.ucl.ac.uk/cls-studies/millennium-cohort-study.

10 Sally Goddard Blythe et al., 'Neuromotor Readiness for School: The Primitive Reflex Status of Young Children at the Start and End of Their First Year at School in the United Kingdom,' *Education 3–13: International Journal of Primary, Elementary and Early Years Education* (2021), https://doi.org/10.1080/03004279.2021.1895276.

11 Goddard Blyth, *The Well Balanced Child*, 41.

12 Jeannette T. Crenshaw, 'Healthy Birth Practice #6: Keep Mother and Baby Together – It's Best for Mother, Baby, and Breastfeeding,' *Journal of Perinatal Education* 23, no. 4 (2014): 211–217, https://doi.org/10.1891/1058-1243.23.4.211.

13 Stefaan W. Verbruggen et al., 'Stresses and Strains on the Human Fetal Skeleton During Development,' *Journal of the Royal Society Interface* 15, no. 138 (January 2018), https://doi.org/10.1098/rsif.2017.0593.

14 'Sudden Infant Death Syndrome (SIDS),' NHS, last modified October 27, 2021, https://www.nhs.uk/conditions/sudden-infant-death-syndrome-sids.

15 World Health Organization, *Guidelines on Physical Activity, Sedentary Behaviour and Sleep for Children Under 5 Years of Age* (Geneva: World Health Organization, 2019), viii, 6.

16 Lyndel Hewitt et al., 'Tummy Time and Infant Health Outcomes: A Systematic Review,' *Pediatrics* 145, no. 6 (June 2020), https://doi.org/10.1542/peds.2019-2168.

17 Michelle Lampl and Michael L. Johnson, 'Infant Growth in Length Follows Prolonged Sleep and Increased Naps,' *Sleep* 34, no. 5 (May 2011): 641–650, https://doi.org/10.1093/sleep/34.5.641.

18 Katy Bowman, *Movement Matters: Essays on Movement Science, Movement Ecology, and the Nature of Movement* (Washington: Propriometrics Press, 2016), 53.

19 Sarah Wong, Louise Ada, and Jane Butler, 'Differences in Ankle Range Of Motion Between Pre-Walking and Walking Infants,' *Australian Journal of Physiotherapy* 44, no. 1 (1998): 57–60, https://doi.org/10.1016/S0004-9514(14)60366-4.

20 B. D. Baggett and G. Young, 'Ankle Joint Dorsiflexion. Establishment of a Normal Range,' *Journal of the American Podiatric Medical Association* 83, no. 5 (May 1993): 251-254.

21 Lexico, s.v. 'joint (n.),' accessed November 12, 2021, https://www.lexico.com/definition/joint; Cambridge Dictionary Online, s.v. 'joint (n.),' accessed November 12, 2021, https://dictionary.cambridge.org/dictionary/english/joint.

22 'Anatomy of a Joint,' Stanford Children's Health, accessed November 12, 2021, https://www.stanfordchildrens.org/en/topic/default?id=anatomy-of-a-joint-85-P00044.

23 David Lesondak, 'Fascia, Tensegrity, and the Cell,' in *Fascia: What It Is and Why It Matters* (Scotland: Handspring Publishing, 2017), 21–40.

24 Whitney G. Cole, Jesse M. Lingeman, and Karen E. Adolph, 'Go Naked: Diapers Affect Infant Walking,' *Developmental Science* 15, no. 6 (November 2012): 783–790, https://doi.org/10.1111/j.1467-7687.2012.01169.x.

25 Jitka Marencakova et al., 'How Do Novice and Improver Walkers Move in Their Home Environments? An Open-Sourced Infant's Gait Video Analysis,' *PLOS ONE* 14, no. 6 (June 2019), https://doi.org/10.1371/journal.pone.0218665.

26 Anthony N. Turner and Ian Jeffreys, 'The Stretch-Shortening Cycle: Proposed Mechanisms and Methods for Enhancement,' *Strength and Conditioning Journal* 32, no. 4 (August 2010): 87–99, https://doi.org/10.1519/SSC.0b013e3181e928f9.

27 Nathaniel J. Dominy, 'Evolution of Sensory Receptor Specializations in the Glabrous Skin,' in *Encyclopedia of Neuroscience*, ed. Larry R. Squire, vol. 4 (London: Academic Press, 2009), 39–42, https://doi.org/10.1016/B978-008045046-9.00956-6.

28 Phil Hoffman, 'Conclusions Drawn from a Comparative Study of the Feet of Barefooted and Shoe-Wearing Peoples,' *The American Journal of Orthopedic Surgery* s2-3, no. 2 (October 1905): 105–136.

29 William Rossi, 'Why Shoes Make "Normal" Gait Impossible,' *Podiatry Management*, March 1999, 50–61.

30 William Rossi, 'Children's Footwear: Launching Site for Adult Foot Ills,' *Podiatry Management,* October 2002, 83–100.

31 Sam Murphy, 'Why Barefoot Is Best for Children,' *Guardian*, August 9, 2010, https://www.theguardian.com/lifeandstyle/2010/aug/09/barefoot-best-for-children.

32 Anita Ellen Williams, 'Special Theme Article: Science and Sociology of Footwear,' *Journal of Foot and Ankle Research* 11, article no. 52 (2018), https://doi.org/10.1186/s13047-018-0293-y.

33 Stewart C. Morrison et al., 'Big Issues for Small Feet: Developmental, Biomechanics and Clinical Narratives on Children's Footwear,' *Journal of Foot and Ankle Research* 11, article no. 39 (2018), https://doi.org/10.1186/s13047-018-0281-2.

34 Caleb Wegener et al., 'Effect of Children's Shoes on Gait: A Systematic Review and Meta-Analysis,' *Journal of Foot and Ankle Research* 4, article no. 3 (2011), https://doi.org/10.1186/1757-1146-4-3.

35 Simone Cranage et al., 'The Impact of Shoe Flexibility on Gait, Pressure and Muscle Activity of Young Children. A Systematic Review,' *Journal of Foot and Ankle Research* 12, article no. 55 (2019), https://doi.org/10.1186/s13047-019-0365-7.

36 Juha-Pekka Kulmala et al., 'Running in Highly Cushioned Shoes Increases Leg Stiffness and Amplifies Impact Loading,' *Scientific Reports* 8, article no. 17496 (November 2018), https://doi.org/10.1038/s41598-018-35980-6.

37 Sarah Shultz et al., 'Metabolic Differences Between Shod and Barefoot Walking in Children,' *International Journal of Sports Medicine* 37, no. 5 (2016): 401–404, https://doi.org/10.1055/s-0035-1569349; Karsten Hollander et al., 'Growing-up (Habitually) Barefoot Influences the Development of Foot and Arch Morphology in Children and Adolescents,' *Scientific Reports* 7, article no. 8079 (2017), https://doi.org/10.1038/s41598-017-07868-4; Astrid Zech et al., 'Motor Skills of Children and Adolescents Are Influenced by Growing Up Barefoot or Shod,' *Frontiers in Pediatrics* 6, article no. 115 (August 2018), https://doi.org/10.3389/fped.2018.00115; Stacey M. Kung et al., 'Kinematic and Kinetic Differences Between Barefoot and Shod Walking in Children,' *Footwear Science* 7, no. 2 (2015): 95–105, https://doi.org/10.1080/19424280.2015.1014066; Karsten Hollander et al., 'Foot Strike Patterns Differ Between Children and Adolescents Growing Up Barefoot vs. Shod,' *International Journal of Sports Medicine* 39, no. 2 (February 2018): 97–103, https://doi.org/10.1055/s-0043-120344.

38 Rossi, 'Children's Footwear,' 83–84

39 Hoffman, 'Conclusions Drawn,' 112.

40 Jenny Wood, 'A Parent's Guide To Buying Toddler Shoes,' *Huffington Post*, October 19, 2016, https://www.huffingtonpost.co.uk/entry/a-parents-guide-to-buying-toddler-shoes_uk_57ab5f28e4b0b3afa75cf376.

41 Cylie Williams et al., 'Soft Soled Footwear Has Limited Impact on Toddler Gait,' *PLOS ONE* 16, no. 5 (May 2021): e0251175, https://doi.org/10.1371/journal.pone.0251175.

42 Irene Davis, 'Benefits of Barefoot/Minimal Footwear and Walking in Adults,' speech recorded as part of The Barefoot Movement Conference hosted by Vivobarefoot on March 30, 2021, YouTube video, https://youtu.be/AYgpDQ2s-dM.

43 Rory Curtis and Kristiaan D'Août, 'Daily Activity in Minimal Footwear Increases Foot Strength,' *Footwear Science* 11, sup. 1 (2019): s151–s152, https://doi.org/10.1080/19424280.2019.1606299.

44 Deborah A. Nawoczenski, Judith F. Baumhauer, and Brian R. Umberger, 'Relationship Between Clinical Measurements and Motion of the First Metatarsophalangeal Joint During Gait,' *The Journal of Bone & Joint Surgery* 81, no. 3 (March 1999): 370–376, https://doi.org/10.2106/00004623-199903000-00009; Steven D. Waldman, 'Functional Anatomy of the Ankle and Foot,' in *Physical Diagnosis of Pain: An Atlas of Signs and Symptoms* (Philadelphia: Elsevier, 2021), 390–392.

45 Angus Chard et al., 'Effect of Thong Style Flip-Flops on Children's Barefoot Walking and Jogging Kinematics,' *Journal of Foot and Ankle Research* 6, article no. 8 (2013), https://doi.org/10.1186/1757-1146-6-8.

46 Jill Ferrari, 'Bunions,' *BMJ Clinical Evidence* (2009): 1112.

47 Nuria K. Mackes et al., 'Early Childhood Deprivation Is Associated with Alterations in Adult Brain Structure Despite Subsequent Environmental Enrichment,' *Proceedings of the National Academy of Sciences* 117, no. 1 (January 2020): 641–649, https://doi.org/10.1073/pnas.1911264116.

48 Abraham Maslow, 'A Theory of Human Motivation,' *Psychological Review* 50, no. 4 (1943): 370–396, https://doi.org/10.1037/h0054346.

49 Tiffany Field et al., 'Cortisol Decreases and Serotonin and Dopamine Increase Following Massage Therapy,' *International Journal of Neuroscience* 115, no. 10 (2005): 1397–1413, https://doi.org/10.1080/00207450590956459.

50 Joshua A. Waxenbaum, Vamsi Reddy; and Matthew Varacallo. *Anatomy, Autonomic Nervous System* (Treasure Island, FL: StatPearls Publishing, 2021), https://www.ncbi.nlm.nih.gov/books/NBK539845.

51 Tiffany Field, 'Enhancing Growth,' in Touch Therapy (London: Churchill Livingstone, 2000), 1–43; Tiffany Field and Miguel Diego, 'Vagal Activity, Early Growth and Emotional Development,' *Infant Behaviour & Development* 31, no. 3 (September 2008): 361–373.

52 Nimet Karatas and Aysegul Isler Dalgic, 'Effects of Reflexology on Child Health: A Systematic Review,' *Complementary Therapies in Medicine* 50, article no. 102364 (May 2020), https://doi.org/10.1016/j.ctim.2020.102364.

BIBLIOGRAPHY AND RECOMMENDED READING

Head to my website for recommended books for extended reading, covering topics such as reflexes, movement, early development and infant massage.

A

Ackerman, Sandra. 'The Development and Shaping of the Brain.' In *Discovering the Brain*, 86–103. Washington: National Academies Press, 1992. https://www.ncbi.nlm.nih.gov/books/NBK234146.

Adolph, Karen E., and John M. Franchak. 'The Development of Motor Behavior.' *WIREs Cognitive Science* 8, no. 1–2 (January–April 2017): e1430. https://doi.org/10.1002/wcs.1430.

Adolph, Karen E., Sarah E. Berger, and Andrew J. Leo. 'Development Continuity? Crawling, Cruising and Walking.' *Developmental Science* 14, no. 2 (March 2011): 306-318. https://doi.org/10.1111/j.1467-7687.2010.00981.x.

Adolph, Karen E., Whitney G. Cole, Meghana Komati, Jessie S. Garciaguirre, Daryaneh Badaly, Jesse M. Lingeman, Gladys L. Y. Chan, and Rachel B. Sotsky. 'How Do You Learn to Walk? Thousands of Steps and Dozens of Falls Per Day.' *Psychological Science* 23, no. 11 (2012): 1387-1394. https://doi.org/10.1177/0956797612446346.

B

Baggett, B. D., and G. Young. 'Ankle Joint Dorsiflexion. Establishment of a Normal Range.' *Journal of the American Podiatric Medical Association* 83, no. 5 (May 1993): 251-254.

Barisch-Fritz, Bettina, and Marlene Mauch. 'Foot Development in Childhood and Adolescence.' In *Handbook of Footwear Design and Manufacture*. Cambridge: Woodhead Publishing Limited, 2013.

Beach, Phillip. *Muscles and Meridians: The Manipulation of Shape*. London: Churchill Livingstone, 2010.

Bertsch, Carola, Heidi Unger, Winfried Winkelmann, and Dieter Rosenbaum. 'Evaluation of Early Walking Patterns from Plantar Pressure Distribution Measurements. First Year Results of 42 Children.' *Gait and Posture* 19, no. 3 (June 2004): 235–242. https://doi.org/10.1016/S0966-6362(03)00064-X.

Blomberg, Harold, and Moira Dempsey. *Movements that Heal: Rhythmic Movement Training and Primitive Reflex Integration*. Sunnybank Hills, QLD: BookPal, 2011.

Blottner, Dieter, Y. Huang, Gabor Trautmann, and L. Sun. 'The Fascia: Continuum Linking Bone and Myofascial Bag for Global and Local Body Movement Control on Earth and in Space. A Scoping Review.' *Reach* 14–15 (June–September 2019). https://doi.org/10.1016/j.reach.2019.100030.

Bojsen-Møller, Finn, and Larry Lamoreux. 'Significance of Free Dorsiflexion of the Toes in Walking.' *Acta Orthopaedica Scandinavica* 50, no. 4 (1979): 471-479. https://doi.org/10.3109/17453677908989792.

Bordoni, Bruno, and Fabiola Marelli. 'Emotions in Motion: Myofascial Interoception.' *Complementary Medicine Research* 24, no. 2 (March 2017): 110-113. https://doi.org/10.1159/000464149.

Bosch, Kerstin, Joachim Gerss, and Dieter Rosenbaum. 'Preliminary Normative Values for Foot Loading Parameters of the Developing Child.' *Gait and Posture* 26, no. 2 (July 2007): 238–247. https://doi.org/10.1016/j.gaitpost.2006.09.014.

Bourne, Matthew, Aditi Talkad, and Matthew Varacallo. 'Anatomy, Bony Pelvis and Lower Limb, Foot Fascia.' *NCBI Bookshelf*. Treasure Island, FL: StatPearls Publishing, 2021. https://www.ncbi.nlm.nih.gov/books/NBK526043.

Bowman, Katy. *Movement Matters: Essays on Movement Science, Movement Ecology, and the Nature of Movement*. Washington: Propriometrics Press, 2016.

Brandes, Bonnie L. *The Symphony of Reflexes: Interventions for Human Development, Autism, ADHD, CP, and Other Neurological Disorders*. North Charleston, SC: Quantum Reflex Integration, Inc, 2015.

Burrow, Gordon, Keith Rome, and Nat Padhiar. *Neale's Disorders of the Foot and Ankle*. 9th ed. London: Elsevier, 2020.

C

Chard, Angus, Andrew Greene, Adrienne Hunt, Benedicte Vanwanseele, and Richard Smith. 'Effect of Thong Style Flip-Flops on Children's Barefoot Walking and Jogging Kinematics.' *Journal of Foot and Ankle Research* 6, article no. 8 (2013). https://doi.org/10.1186/1757-1146-6-8.

Centre for Longitudinal Studies, University College London. 'Millennium Cohort Study.' Last modified 26 October, 2021. https://cls.ucl.ac.uk/cls-studies/millennium-cohort-study.

Cerritelli, Francesco, Piero Chiacchiaretta, Francesco Gambi, and Antonio Ferretti. 'Effect of Continuous Touch on Brain Functional Connectivity is Modified by the Operator's Tactile Attention.' *Frontiers in Human Neuroscience* 11, article no. 368 (July 2017). https://doi.org/10.3389/fnhum.2017.00368.

Cole, Whitney G., Jesse M. Lingeman, and Karen E. Adolph. 'Go Naked: Diapers Affect Infant Walking.' *Developmental Science* 15, no. 6 (November 2012): 783–790. https://doi.org/10.1111/j.1467-7687.2012.01169.x.

Cowgill, Libby W., Anna Warrener, Herman Pontzer, and Cara Ocobock. 'Waddling and Toddling: The Biomechanics Effects of an Immature Gait.' *American Journal of Physical Anthropology* 143, no. 1 (September 2010): 52-61. https://doi.org/10.1002/ajpa.21289.

Cranage, Simone, Luke Perraton, Kelly-Ann Bowles, and Cylie Williams. 'The Impact of Shoe Flexibility on Gait, Pressure and Muscle Activity of Young Children. A Systematic Review.' *Journal of Foot and Ankle Research* 12, article no. 55 (2019). https://doi.org/10.1186/s13047-019-0365-7.

Crenshaw, Jeannette T. 'Healthy Birth Practice #6: Keep Mother and Baby Together – It's Best for Mother, Baby, and Breastfeeding.' *Journal of Perinatal Education* 23, no. 4 (2014): 211–217. https://doi.org/10.1891/1058-1243.23.4.211.

Crucianelli, Laura, and Mara Laura Filippetti. 'Developmental Perspectives on Interpersonal Affective Touch.' *Topoi* 39 (2020): 575–586. https://doi.org/10.1007/s11245-018-9565-1.

Curtis, Rory, and Kristiaan D'Août. 'Daily Activity in Minimal Footwear Increases Foot Strength.' *Footwear Science* 11, sup. 1 (2019): s151–s152. https://doi.org/10.1080/19424280.2019.1606299.

Czerwinski, Florian, Ewa Tomasik, and Aldona Mahaczek-Kordowska. 'The Ossification of Tarsal Bones and Distal End of Tibia in Human Foetus.' *Folia Morphologica* 60, no. 3 (2001): 195-198.

D

Davis, Irene. 'Benefits of Barefoot/Minimal Footwear and Walking in Adults.' The Barefoot Movement Conference hosted by Vivobarefoot. March 30, 2021, YouTube video. https://youtu.be/AYgpDQ2s-dM.

Dempsey, Moira. *Beyond the Sea Squirt: A Journey with Reflexes*. Melbourne: Beyond the Sea Squirt Publications, 2019.

Dewolf, Arthur Henri, Francesca Sylos-Labini, Germana Cappellini, Francesco Lacquaniti, and Yury Ivanenko. 'Emergence of Different Gaits in Infancy: Relationship Between Developing Neural Circuitries and Changing Biomechanics' *Frontiers in Bioengineering and Biotechnology* 8, article no. 473 (May 2020). https://doi.org/10.3389/fbioe.2020.00473.

Dominici, Nadia, Yuri P. Ivanenko, Germana Cappellini, Maria Luisa Zampagni, Francesco Lacquaniti. 'Kinematic Strategies in Newly Walking Toddlers Stepping Over Different Support Surfaces.' *Journal of Neurophysiology* 103, no. 3 (March 2010): 1673–1684. https://doi.org/10.1152/jn.00945.2009.

Dominy, Nathaniel J. 'Evolution of Sensory Receptor Specializations in the Glabrous Skin.' Vol. 4 of *Encyclopedia of Neuroscience*, edited by Larry R. Squire, 39–42. London: Academic Press, 2009. https://doi.org/10.1016/B978-008045046-9.00956-6.

E

Earls, James. *Born to Walk, Myofascial Efficiency and the Body in Movement.* Chichester: Lotus Publishing, 2014.

Evans, Angela M. 'Mitigating Clinician and Community Concerns About Children's Flatfeet, Intoning Gait, Knock Knees or Bow Legs.' *Journal of Paediatrics and Child Health* 53, no. 11 (November 2017): 1050-1053. https://doi.org/10.1111/jpc.13761.

F

Field, Tiffany. 'Enhancing Growth.' In *Touch Therapy*, 1–43. London: Churchill Livingstone, 2000.

Field, Tiffany, Maria Hernandez-Reif, Miguel Diego, Saul Schanberg, and Cynthia Kuhn. 'Cortisol Decreases and Serotonin and Dopamine Increase Following Massage Therapy.' *International Journal of Neuroscience* 115, no. 10 (2005): 1397–1413. https://doi.org/10.1080/00207450590956459.

Field, Tiffany, and Miguel Diego. 'Vagal Activity, Early Growth and Emotional Development.' *Infant Behavior & Development* 31, no. 3 (September 2008): 361–373. https://www.doi.org/10.1016/j.infbeh.2007.12.008.

G

Goddard Blythe, Sally. *Neuromotor Immaturity in Children and Adults.* Chichester: Wiley Blackwell, 2014.

Goddard Blythe, Sally. *Raising Happy Healthy Children. Why Mothering Matters.* Gloucestershire, UK: Hawthorn Press, 2017.

Goddard Blythe, Sally. *The Well Balanced Child: Movement and Early Learning.* Gloucestershire: Hawthorn Press, 2005.

Goddard Blythe, Sally, Rebecca Duncombe, Pat Preedy, and Trish Gorely. 'Neuromotor Readiness for School: The Primitive Reflex Status of Young Children at the Start and End of Their First Year at School in the United Kingdom.' *Education 3–13: International Journal of Primary, Elementary and Early Years Education* (2021). https://doi.org/10.1080/03004279.2021. 1895276.

Graven, Stanley N., and Joy V. Browne. 'Sensory Development in the Fetus, Neonate, and Infant: Introduction and Overview.' *Newborn and Infant Nursing Reviews* 8, no. 4 (December 2008): 169–172. https://doi.org/10.1053/j. nainr.2008.10.007.

H

Hallemans, Ann, Dirk De Clercq, Stefaan Van Dongen, and Peter Aerts. 'Changes in Foot-Function Parameters During the First 5 Months After the Onset of Independent Walking: A Longitudinal Follow-Up Study.' *Gait and Posture* 23, no. 2 (February 2006): 142–148. https://doi.org/10.1016/j. gaitpost.2005.01.003.

Hanscom, Angela J. *Balanced and Barefoot: How Unrestricted Outdoor Play Makes for Strong, Confident, and Capable Children.* Oakland, CA: New Harbinger Publications, 2016.

Hewitt, Lyndel, Erin Kerr, Rebecca M. Stanley, and Anthony D. Okely. 'Tummy Time and Infant Health Outcomes: A Systematic Review.' *Pediatrics* 145, no. 6 (June 2020). https://doi.org/10.1542/peds.2019-2168.

Hodgson, Lisa, Charlotte Grwocott, Anita Williams, Chris Nester, and Stewart C. Morrison. 'Finding Top Tips for Tiny Toes: A Thematic Analysis of Internet Based Information About Children's Foot Health.' *Association of Paediatric Chartered Physiotherapists Journal* 11, no. 1 (June 2020): 17–24.

Hodgson, Lisa, Molly Hodges, Anita. E. Williams, Christ Nester, and Stewart C. Morrison. 'The "Price-Tag" of Foot Health in Infancy and Early Childhood: A Cross Sectional Survey of UK Parents.' *European Journal of Pediatrics* 180, no. 4 (2021): 1561–1570. https://doi.org/10.1007/s00431-020-03920-0.

Hoffman, Phil. 'Conclusions Drawn from a Comparative Study of the Feet of Barefooted and Shoe-Wearing Peoples.' *The American Journal of Orthopedic Surgery* s2-3, no. 2 (October 1905): 105–136.

Hollander, Karsten, Johanna Elsabe de Villiers, Susanne Sehner, Karl Wegscheider, Klaus-Michael Braumann, Ranel Venter, and Astrid Zech.

'Growing-up (Habitually) Barefoot Influences the Development of Foot and Arch Morphology in Children and Adolescents.' *Scientific Reports* 7, article no. 8079 (2017). https://doi.org/10.1038/s41598-017-07868-4

Hollander, Karsten, Johanna Elsabe de Villiers, Ranel Venter, Susanne Sehner, Karl Wegscheider, Klaus-Michael Braumann, and Astrid Zech. 'Foot Strike Patterns Differ Between Children and Adolescents Growing Up Barefoot vs. Shod.' *International Journal of Sports Medicine* 39, no. 2 (February 2018): 97–103. https://doi.org/10.1055/s-0043-120344.

Hoogenboom, Barbara, and Michael L. Voight. 'Rolling Revisited: Using Rolling to Assess and Treat Neuromuscular Control and Coordination of the Core and Extremities of Athletes.' *The International Journal of Sports Physical Therapy* 10, no. 6 (November 2015): 787–802.

Howell, Daniel. *The Barefoot Book. 50 Great Reasons to Kick Off Your Shoes.* Alameda, CA: Hunter House, 2010.

I

Idris, Ferial Hadipoetro. 'The Growth of Foot Arches and Influencing Factors.' *Paediatric Indonesiana* 45, no. 3 (2005). https://doi.org/10.14238/pi45.3. 2005.111-7.

J

Jones, Martha Wilson. 'Supine and Prone Infant Positioning: A Winning Combination.' *The Journal of Perinatal Education* 13, no. 1 (2004): 10-20. https://doi.org/10.1624/105812404X109357.

K

Karatas, Nimet, and Aysegul Isler Dalgic. 'Effects of Reflexology on Child Health: A Systematic Review.' *Complementary Therapies in Medicine* 50, article no. 102364 (May 2020). https://doi.org/10.1016/j.ctim.2020.102364.

Kulmala, Juha-Pekka, Jukka Kosonen, Jussi Nurminen, and Janne Avela. 'Running in Highly Cushioned Shoes Increases Leg Stiffness and Amplifies Impact Loading.' *Scientific Reports* 8, article no. 17496 (November 2018). https://doi.org/10.1038/s41598-018-35980-6.

Kung, Stacey M., Philip W. Fink, Patria Hume, and Sarah P. Shultz. 'Kinematic and Kinetic Differences Between Barefoot and Shod Walking in Children.' *Footwear Science* 7, no. 2 (2015): 95–105. https://doi.org/10.1080/19424280.2015.1014066.

L

Lampl, Michelle, and Michael L. Johnson. 'Infant Growth in Length Follows Prolonged Sleep and Increased Naps.' *Sleep* 34, no. 5 (May 2011): 641–650. https://doi.org/10.1093/sleep/34.5.641.

Leboyer, Frederick. *Loving Hands: The Traditional Art of Baby Massage.* New York: Newmarket Press, 1976.

Lesondak, David. *Fascia: What It Is and Why It Matters.* Scotland: Handspring Publishing, 2017.

M

Maffetone, Phil. 'Ticking Time Bomb: Children's Shoes Cause Health Problems Later in Life for Adults.' Last modified April 30, 2015. https://philmaffetone. com/kids-shoes.

Marencakova, Jitka, Carina Price, Tomas Maly, Frantisek Zahalka, and Christopher Nester. 'How Do Novice and Improver Walkers Move in Their Home Environments? An Open-Sourced Infant's Gait Video Analysis.' *PLOS ONE* 14, no. 6 (June 2019). https://doi.org/10.1371/journal.pone.0218665.

Marshall, Andrew G., Manohar L. Sharma, Kate Marley K, Hakan Olausson, and Francis P. McGlone. 'Spinal signaling of C-fiber mediated pleasant touch in humans.' *eLife* 8 (December 2019): e51642. https://doi.org/10.1101/780635.

Martín-Alguacil, Nieves, Ignacio de Gaspar, Justine M. Schober, and Donald W. Pfaff. 'Somatosensation: End Organs for Tactile Sensation.' In *Neuroscience in the 21st Century,* edited by Donald W. Pfaff, 743–780. Springer, New York: Springer, 2013. https://doi.org/10.1007/978-1-4614-1997-6_27.

Maslow, Abraham. 'A Theory of Human Motivation.' *Psychological Review* 50, no. 4 (1943): 370–396. https://doi.org/10.1037/h0054346.

McClure, Vimala. *Infant Massage: A Handbook for Loving Parents.* 4th ed. New York: Bantam Books, 2017.

Moore, Keith L., T. V. N Persaud, and Mark G. Torchia. *The Developing Human: Clinically Orientated Embryology.* 11th ed. Philadelphia: Elsevier, 2020.

Morrison, Stewart C., Carina Price, Juliet McClymont, and Chris Nester. 'Big Issues for Small Feet: Developmental, Biomechanics and Clinical Narratives on Children's Footwear.' *Journal of Foot and Ankle Research* 11, article no. 39 (2018). https://doi.org/10.1186/s13047-018-0281-2.

Morrison, Stewart C., Juliet McClymont, Carina Price, and Chris Nester. 'Time to Revise Our Dialogue: How *Flat* is the Paediatric *Flat*foot?' *Journal of*

Foot and Ankle Research 10, article no. 50 (2017). https://doi.org/10.1186/s13047-017-0233-2.

Murphy, Sam. 'Why Barefoot Is Best for Children.' *Guardian*, August 9, 2010. https://www.theguardian.com/lifeandstyle/2010/aug/09/barefoot-best-for-children.

N

Nawoczenski, Deborah A., Judith F. Baumhauer, and Brian R. Umberger. 'Relationship Between Clinical Measurements and Motion of the First Metatarsophalangeal Joint During Gait.' *The Journal of Bone & Joint Surgery* 81, no. 3 (March 1999): 370–376. https://doi.org/10.2106/00004623-199903000-00009.

Nguyen, John D., and Hieu Duong. *Neurosurgery, Sensory Homunculus.* Treasure Island, FL: StatPearls Publishing, 2021. https://www.ncbi.nlm.nih.gov/books/NBK549841.

NHS. 'Sudden Infant Death Syndrome (SIDS).' Last modified October 27, 2021. https://www.nhs.uk/conditions/sudden-infant-death-syndrome-sids.

Mackes, Nuria K., Dennis Golm, Sagari Sarkar, Robert Kumsta, Michael Rutter, Graeme Fairchild, Mitul A. Mehta, and Edmund J. S. Sonuga-Barke. 'Early Childhood Deprivation Is Associated with Alterations in Adult Brain Structure Despite Subsequent Environmental Enrichment.' *Proceedings of the National Academy of Sciences* 117, no. 1 (January 2020): 641–649. https://doi.org/10.1073/pnas.1911264116.

P

Price, Carina, Juliet McClymont, Farina Hashmi, Stewart C. Morrison, and Christopher Nester. 'Development of the Infant Foot as a Load Bearing Structure: Study Protocol for a Longitudinal Evaluation (the Small Steps Study).' *Journal of Foot and Ankle Research* 11, no. 33 (December 2018). https://doi.org/10.1186/s13047-018-0273-2.

Price, Carina, Stewart C. Morrison, Farina Hashmi, Jill Phethean, and Christopher Nester. 'Biomechanics of the Infant Foot During the Transition to Independent Walking: A Narrative Review.' *Gait and Posture* 59 (January 2018): 140–146. https://doi.org/10.1016/j.gaitpost.2017.09.005.

R

Rendle-Short, John. 'Normal and Abnormal Development in Babies.' *Australian Journal of Physiotherapy* 8, no. 3 (December 1962): 103–107. https://doi.org/10.1016/S0004-9514(14)60781-9.

Rossi, William. 'Children's Footwear: Launching Site for Adult Foot Ills.' *Podiatry Management*, October 2002, 83–100.

Rossi, William. 'Why Shoes Make "Normal" Gait Impossible.' *Podiatry Management*, March 1999, 50–61.

S

Samson, William, Bruno Dohin, Guillaume Desroches, Jean-Luc Chaverot, Raphaël Dumas, and Laurence Cheze. 'Foot Mechanics During the First Six Years of Independent Walking.' *Journal of Biomechanics* 44, no. 7 (April 2011): 1321–1327. https://doi.org/10.1016/j.jbiomech.2011.01.007.

Schleip, Robert, Thomas W. Findley, Leon Chaitow, and Peter A. Huijing, eds. *Fascia: The Tensional Network of the Human Body*. London: Churchill Livingstone, 2012.

Schleip, Robert. 'Innervation of Fascia.' In *Fascia, Function, and Medical Applications*, edited by David Lesondak and Angeli Maun Akey, 61–70. Boca Raton: CRC Press, 2021.

Shultz, Sarah, S. D. Houltham, Stacey Kung, and Patria Hume. 'Metabolic Differences Between Shod and Barefoot Walking in Children.' *International Journal of Sports Medicine* 37, no. 5 (2016): 401–404. https://doi.org/10.1055/s-0035-1569349.

Stanojevic, Milan. 'Neonatal Aspects: Is There Continuity?' *Donald School Journal of Ultrasound in Obstetrics and Gynecology* 6, no. 2 (2012):189-196. https://doi.org/10.5005/jp-journals-10009-1242.

Strach, E. H. 'Club-Foot Through the Centuries.' In *Historical Aspects of Pediatric Surgery*, edited by Peter Paul Rickham, 215–237. Vol. 20 of *Progress in Pediatric Surgery*. Berlin: Springer, 1986. https://doi.org/10.1007/978-3-642-70825-1_16.

T

Tickle, Cheryll. 'How the Embryo Makes a Limb: Determination, Polarity and Identity.' *Journal of Anatomy* 227, no. 4. (October 2015): 418-430. https://doi.org/10.1111/joa.12361.

Trinkaus, Erik, and Hong Shang. 'Anatomical Evidence for the Antiquity of Human Footwear: Tianyuan and Sunghir.' *Journal of Archaeological Science* 35, no. 7 (July 2008): 1928–1933. https://doi.org/10.1016/j.jas.2007.12.002.

Turner, Anthony N., and Ian Jeffreys. 'The Stretch-Shortening Cycle: Proposed Mechanisms and Methods for Enhancement.' *Strength and Conditioning Journal* 32, no. 4 (August 2010): 87–99. https://doi.org/10.1519/SSC.0b013e3181e928f9.

Turner, Claire, Matthew D. Gardiner, Ann Midgley, and Anastasia Stefanis. 'A Guide to the Management of Paediatric Pes Planus.' *Australian Journal of General Practice* 49, no. 5 (May 2020). https://doi.org/10.31128/AJGP-09-19-5089.

Turner, Warren, and Linda Merriman. *Clinical Skills in Treating the Foot.* 2nd ed. London: Churchill Livingstone, 2005.

V

Verbruggen, Stefaan W., Bernhard Kainz, Susan C. Shelmerdine, Joseph V. Hajnal, Mary A. Rutherford, Owen J. Arthurs, Andrew T. M. Phillips, and Niamh C. Nowlan. 'Stresses and Strains on the Human Fetal Skeleton During Development.' *Journal of the Royal Society Interface* 15, no. 138 (January 2018). https://doi.org/10.1098/rsif.2017.0593.

Viseux, Frederic J. F. 'The Sensory Role of the Sole of the Foot: Review and Update on Clinical Perspectives.' *Neurophysiologie Clinique* 50, no. 1 (February 2020): 55–68. https://doi.org/10.1016/jneucli.2019.12.003.

W

Waldman, Steven D. 'Functional Anatomy of the Ankle and Foot.' in *Physical Diagnosis of Pain: An Atlas of Signs and Symptoms*, 390–392. Philadelphia: Elsevier, 2021.

Waxenbaum, Joshua A., Vamsi Reddy; and Matthew Varacallo. *Anatomy, Autonomic Nervous System.* Treasure Island, FL: StatPearls Publishing, 2021. https://www.ncbi.nlm.nih.gov/books/NBK539845/.

Wegener, Caleb, Adrienne E. Hunt, Benedicte Vanwanseele, Joshua Burns, and Richard M. Smith. 'Effect of Children's Shoes on Gait: A Systematic Review and Meta-Analysis.' *Journal of Foot and Ankle Research* 4, article no. 3 (2011). https://doi.org/10.1186/1757-1146-4-3.

Wikler, Simon J. 'Preventing Children's Foot Trouble.' In *Take Off Your Shoes and Walk.* New York: Devin-Adair Co, 1961. http://www.unshod.org/pfbc/swc5.htm.

Williams, Anita Ellen. 'Special Theme Article: Science and Sociology of Footwear.' *Journal of Foot and Ankle Research* 11, article no. 52 (2018). https://doi.org/10.1186/s13047-018-0293-y.

Williams, Cylie, Jessica Kolic, Wen Wu, and Kade Paterson. 'Soft Soled Footwear Has Limited Impact on Toddler Gait.' *PLOS ONE* 16, no. 5 (May 2021): e0251175. https://doi.org/10.1371/journal.pone.0251175.

Whitehead, Kimberley, Judith Meek, and Lorenzo Fabrizi. 'Developmental Trajectory of Movement-Related Cortical Oscillations During Active Sleep in a Cross-Sectional Cohort of Pre-Term and Full-Term Human Infants.' *Scientific Reports* 8, article no. 17516 (2018). https://doi.org/10.1038/s41598-018-35850-1.

Wong, Sarah, Louise Ada, and Jane Butler. 'Differences in Ankle Range Of Motion Between Pre-Walking and Walking Infants.' *Australian Journal of Physiotherapy* 44, no. 1 (1998): 57–60. https://doi.org/10.1016/S0004-9514(14)60366-4.

Wood, Jenny. 'A Parent's Guide To Buying Toddler Shoes.' *Huffington Post*, October 19, 2016. https://www.huffingtonpost.co.uk/entry/a-parents-guide-to-buying-toddler-shoes_uk_57ab5f28e4b0b3afa75cf37.

World Health Organization. *Guidelines on Physical Activity, Sedentary Behaviour and Sleep for Children Under 5 Years of Age.* Geneva: World Health Organization, 2019. https://apps.who.int/iris/handle/10665/311664.

World Health Organization. *Monitoring Children's Development in the Primary Care Services: Moving from a Focus on Child Deficits to Family-Centred Participatory Support. Report of a Virtual Technical Meeting, 9–10 June 2020.* Geneva: World Health Organization, 2020. https://www.who.int/publications/i/item/9789240012479.

Z

Zech, Astrid, Ranel Venter, Johanna E. de Villiers, Susanne Sehner, Karl Wenscheider, and Karsten Hollander. 'Motor Skills of Children and Adolescents Are Influenced by Growing Up Barefoot or Shod.' *Frontiers in Pediatrics* 6, article no. 115 (August 2018). https://doi.org/10.3389/fped.2018.00115.

QUICK REFERENCE GUIDE

QR CODES

ACKNOWLEDGEMENTS

To all my clients, parents and babies who have generously shared their bodies, lives, joys and ailments with me over the last two decades.

To all my teachers of the human body, there is a piece of everyone in here.

To Sue Adstrum who planted the seed, and Samantha Sainsbury for taking my jumbled Lego box of words and sorting it into colours so I could build this book with clarity.

To my mum, Cynthia, for her creativity and help with the images.

To Alicia Bennett, Carly Macleay, Katja Bartsch and Sue Campbell who took the time to read the jumbled words and Peggy Dawson who devoured my words guiding me gently to explore and discover more.

To James Earls, author of *Born to Walk* and *Understanding the Human Foot*, for taking the time to read and provide detailed comments, encouraging and advising me as an expert in the human foot and body.

My heartfelt thanks to the team at Indie Experts for their work behind the scenes, especially Dixie Maria Carlton for her mentoring and guidance and Anne-Marie Tripp for taking my Lego creation to a whole other level.

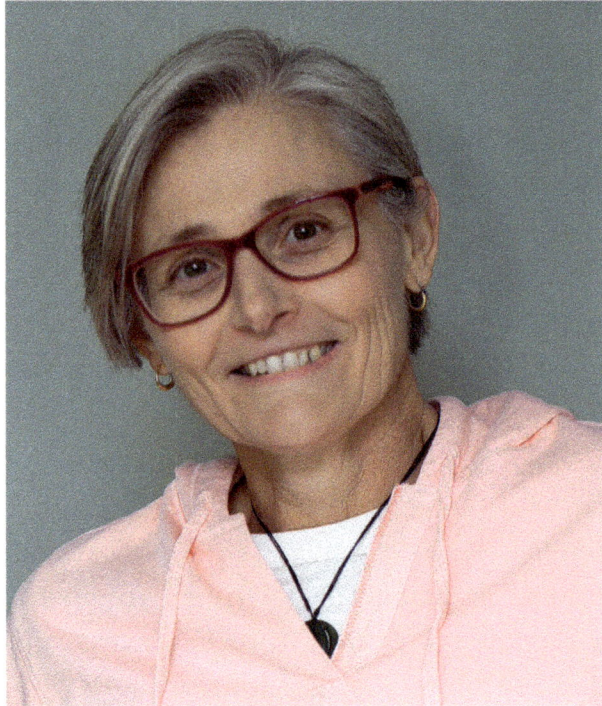

ABOUT BERNIE LANDELS

As an internationally-certified Infant Massage Instructor (IAIM) since 2002, Bernie Landels has helped many parents build strong connections with and foundations for their children through touch and education.

Bernie's journey into working with the body began in 1996 at the New Zealand College of Massage (NZCM), where she gained a Bachelor of Health Studies (Massage and Neuromuscular Therapy). She went on to teach clinical massage at the NZCM from 1999 while also working in private practice, before becoming the owner and director of the college until 2011.

Bernie is passionate about enabling people to gain insight and knowledge about their anatomy to help their own health and wellbeing. Since moving to the UK, Bernie has continued her studies and gained additional qualifications to further understand anatomy, movement and the human form.

While working with adults presenting with pain and postural 'issues', and teaching parents about their infants Bernie started asking the question – what if the 'issues' started developing in the earliest years? This burning question was the catalyst for Bernie to embark on writing *Finding Their Feet:* an accessible and practical guide designed for parents and carers, to equip them for the most important role they will have – guiding their child's development.

'I wish I knew what I know now when my boys were little, they may not have had some of the challenges they faced.' **BERNIE LANDELS**

Based on Bernie's empowering approach, *Finding Their Feet* will build your confidence and provide practical activities for you to experience with your baby, playing, building bonds and foundations for life.

Bernie is a new empty-nester, with two grown-up young sons now exploring the world. She continues to work in private practice in Oxford, UK, working with all ages but focusing on pregnancy massage and sharing the joys of infant massage.

To learn more about Bernie and her work, please visit
https://www.bernielandels.com

www.ingramcontent.com/pod-product-compliance
Lightning Source LLC
Chambersburg PA
CBHW051618030426

42334CB00030B/3246